PERIMENOPAUSE

PERIMENOPAUSE

Edited by

Joseph M. Novi
Riverside Methodist Hospital
Columbus, Ohio, USA

Helen L. Ross
University of Florida College of Medicine
Gainesville, Florida, USA

informa
healthcare

New York   London

Informa Healthcare USA, Inc.
52 Vanderbilt Avenue
New York, NY 10017

© 2009 by Informa Healthcare USA, Inc.
Informa Healthcare is an Informa business

No claim to original U.S. Government works
Printed in the United States of America on acid-free paper
10 9 8 7 6 5 4 3 2 1

International Standard Book Number-10: 0-8247-5449-2 (Hardcover)
International Standard Book Number-13: 978-0-8247-5449-5 (Hardcover)

Library of Congress Cataloging-in-Publication Data

Perimenopause / edited by Joseph M. Novi, Helen L. Ross.
    p. ; cm.
  Includes bibliographical references and index.
  ISBN-13: 978-0-8247-5449-5 (hardcover : alk. paper)
  ISBN-10: 0-8247-5449-2 (hardcover : alk. paper) 1. Perimenopause. I. Novi, Joseph M. II. Ross, Helen L., 1960-
    [DNLM: 1. Perimenopause. WP 580 P4445 2008]
  RG188.P47 2008
  618.1'75--dc22

                                                                              2008025093

For Corporate Sales and Reprint Permissions call 212-520-2700 or write to: Sales Department, 52 Vanderbilt Avenue, 7th floor, New York, NY 10017.

Visit the Informa Web site at
www.informa.com

and the Informa Healthcare Web site at
www.informahealthcare.com

Preface

Perimenopause, the transition from reproductive activity through the menopause, may encompass an entire decade of a woman's life. Dramatic changes take place during these years that set the stage for a woman's health into her older age. While much attention is focused on women in the reproductive years and after menopause, relatively little consideration is given to the perimenopausal transition.

All women who live long enough will experience perimenopause, making this an essential focus of the attention of any practitioner who treats women. We hope that the concepts presented in this textbook will result in your improved understanding of perimenopause and, ultimately, improved care of our patients.

The idea for this book began more than five years ago. We were interested in furnishing the practicing medical care provider with current information regarding this important era in a woman's life. We've tried to provide a broad obstetric and gynecologic view of perimenopause, its symptoms, challenges, and management.

The beginning chapters deal with common problems and questions that perimenopausal women and their healthcare providers encounter frequently. These include complimentary and alternative medicines, abnormal uterine bleeding, and fertility issues. Each chapter presents these issues in the scope of the woman approaching the transition into menopause, highlighting treatment regimens that are specific to this group of women.

The middle portion of the book encompasses the most daunting issues facing the perimenopausal woman; namely, hysterectomy, obstetrical issues, and sexuality. Each of these concerns may have a profound effect on a woman's life, and each has its own management points specific to the perimenopausal woman. The final chapters focus on common urogynecologic complaints: urinary incontinence, pelvic organ prolapse, and fecal incontinence.

The creation of this book has been at times both stimulating and exhausting. We believe that the final product has been worth the effort, and we think you'll agree.

We are deeply indebted to the contributors to this book who have dedicated their lives to improving the quality of medical care for women.

Joseph M. Novi, D.O.
Helen L. Ross, M.D.

Contents

Contributors

Karen L. Hall Department of Community Health and Family Medicine, University of Florida College of Medicine, Gainesville, Florida, U.S.A.

Shae Graham Kosch Behavioral Medicine Program, Department of Community Health and Family Medicine, University of Florida College of Medicine, Gainesville, Florida, U.S.A.

Frederick W. McLean Department of Obstetrics and Gynecology, University of Florida College of Medicine, Gainesville, Florida, U.S.A.

Gina M. Northington Department of Obstetrics and Gynecology, University of Pennsylvania, Philadelphia, Pennsylvania, U.S.A.

Joseph M. Novi Department of Urogynecology and Reconstructive Pelvic Surgery, Riverside Methodist Hospital, Columbus, Ohio, U.S.A.

Douglas S. Richards Department of Obstetrics and Gynecology, University of Florida College of Medicine, Gainesville, Florida, U.S.A.

Alice S. Rhoton-Vlasak Division of Reproductive Endocrinology and Infertility, Department of Obstetrics and Gynecology, University of Florida College of Medicine, Gainesville, Florida, U.S.A.

Emily Saks Department of Obstetrics and Gynecology, University of Pennsylvania, Philadelphia, Pennsylvania, U.S.A.

Judith S. Simms-Cendan Department of Obstetrics and Gynecology, University of Florida College of Medicine, Gainesville, Florida, U.S.A.

I. Keith Stone Department of Obstetrics and Gynecology, University of Florida College of Medicine, Gainesville, Florida, U.S.A.

R. Stan Williams Department of Obstetrics and Gynecology, University of Florida College of Medicine, Gainesville, Florida, U.S.A.

1

Complementary and Alternative Medicine in the Perimenopause

Judith S. Simms-Cendan
Department of Obstetrics and Gynecology, University of Florida College of Medicine, Gainesville, Florida, U.S.A.

I. INTRODUCTION

For many women the transition through the perimenopausal years evolves smoothly. Other women experience a disturbing variety of physical and psychological symptoms. While some seek help from physicians, psychiatrists, and other mainstream providers, a growing number of women are seeking relief outside the purview of conventional medicine. The following discussion addresses the reasons women seek alternative therapies and examines available data regarding benefits and risks of those approaches. The intent is to provide a guide for open discussion between the health care provider and patient regarding use of alternative therapies for symptom relief.

A. Defining Complementary and Alternative Medicine

In order to quantitate the number of women using a complementary and alternative medicine (CAM), it is important first to define CAM. The National Center for Complementary and Alternative Medicine (NCCAM), under the auspices of the National Institutes of Health (NIH), defines CAM as "a group of diverse medical and health care systems, practices, and products that are not presently considered to be part of conventional medicine." Complementary medicine refers to therapy used in conjunction with conventional medicine, while alternative medicine is used in place of conventional treatment.

A myriad of CAM therapies exist. Frequently, CAM therapies are classified by type. Alternative medical systems include homeopathic medicine, traditional Chinese medicine, and Ayurveda.

These systems incorporate alternative theories of human physiology and origins of disease with corresponding treatments. Biologically based theories include herbal products, vitamins, and other naturally occurring substances to treat symptoms and illnesses. Maripulche and body-based methods include massage and chiropractic therapies.

Energy therapy, often used in traditional Chinese medicine systems, includes acupuncture and Reiki. Finally, mind–body interventions are designed to enhance the mind's ability to improve and enhance bodily function. The use of prayer, meditation, and creative expression through art and music has long accompanied conventional medicine.

B. Demographics

Women aged 35 to 49 years comprise the largest consumers of CAM (1). Approximately 50% of perimenopausal women report the use of CAM in the past 12 months, according to the 1997 national survey. The most commonly used modalities include relaxation techniques, herbal therapies, massage, and chiropractic techniques.

A more recently published telephone survey of 886 women aged 45 to 65 years documented an even higher level of use. Seventy-six percent reported use of any therapy; 37% used over-the-counter botanicals, 31% chiropractic, 30% massage therapy, 10% acupuncture, and 9.4% homeopathy. Twenty-two percent of women used alternative therapies specifically for management of menopausal symptoms, and from 89% to 100% found them to be somewhat or very helpful. Among users of conventional hormone replacement therapy (HRT), 8.1% also reported use of alternative therapies such as homeopathic or herbal medicines to manage menopausal symptoms (2).

The reasons perimenopausal women choose CAM therapies are complex and numerous. The underlying driving forces are the inadequacies of the current health care system in the United States, combined with an increasing autonomy in health management, plus expanding availability of sources of CAM.

Perimenopausal women who present to conventional health care providers often report symptoms of fatigue, mood swings, depression, and/or anxiety. In most modern practices, office visits are limited to 15 minutes or less, and evaluation and treatment is limited to laboratory studies and prescription medicines. Psychosocial issues usually are addressed by separate providers, if at all. Traditional medicine systems such as Ayurvedic medicine tend to a more holistic approach. Additionally, traditional practitioners generally spend much more time with patients, providing needed emotional support.

Americans have become increasingly disappointed with the inability of science to find answers to chronic illnesses and symptoms. The well-publicized withdrawal of numerous pharmaceuticals due to adverse effects has heightened the public suspicion of prescription medicine. Most recently, discontinuation of the estrogen/progestin arm of the Women's Health Initiative trial due to the increased risk of breast cancer, pulmonary embolus, and congestive heart disease has fueled fears about use of hormone replacement therapy (3). In fact, the NCCAM responded to the release of well study results with a website cautioning the reflex use of CAM by women discontinuing hormone replacement therapy.

After completion of childbearing, many women decrease the frequency of visits to health care providers. Increased consumer awareness of herbal remedies, combined with ready availability in supermarkets and drug stores, has led to increased use of these products. Sold often on the same shelves are vitamins, there is little regulation of the safety or production consistency of food supplements. Women turn to those products claiming to promote weight loss, enhanced energy, or improved libido in an effort to find a quick fix.

Finally, women also use CAM for real or perceived cost benefits. Many Americans remain uninsured. Office visits and laboratory/radiologic studies continue to spiral upward in cost. Simultaneously, consumer spending on CAM has increased 69% since 1989 with out-of-pocket expenditures for CAM services equaling expenditures for physician services (1,4). Consumer pressure is increasing insurance coverage of CAM services, and providers are being encouraged to refer patients to these services.

Table 1 Summary of CAM Physician Practice Guidelines of the Federation of State Medical Boards

1) Evaluate safety and efficacy of treatments
2) Document history and physical prior to recommendation
3) Document discussion of risk/benefit ratio compared with other treatments
4) Refer to only licensed or state-regulated practitioners
5) Maintain periodic review of results

C. Guidelines for Use of CAM in Medical Practice

In April 2002, the Federation of State Medical Boards of the United States established guidelines for incorporating CAM into medical practice. Essentially, the standards recognized for conventional medicine are applied to CAM. Physicians who prescribe either botanical/herbal treatments or refer to other CAM practitioners are held responsible for monitoring patient outcomes (5).

Section I of the guidelines states that physicians are expected to discriminate between the following types of therapy, whether conventional or CAM:

a) Treatments that are effective and safe, with adequate scientific evidence to support their use.
b) Treatments that are effective, but with some real or potential adverse effects.
c) Treatments that are inadequately studied for efficacy, but have adequate safety data, and
d) Treatments known to be ineffective and dangerous.

Of note, use of CAM itself does not constitute unprofessional behavior (5)

Section II of the guidelines defines conventional and CAM as described earlier in this article. Section III outlines specific physician responsibility. Expected documentation includes a thorough patient evaluation and diagnosis. Diagnostic tests must conform to conventional safety standards. Treatment plans must include documentation of risks and benefits of the proposed therapies. Physicians are expected to refer only to licensed or state-regulated practitioners of CAM. Finally, it is the physician's responsibility to document periodic review of treatment results. Inherent in these recommendations is the assumption that physicians maintain an adequate level of education regarding any recommended therapies.

D. Botanical Therapy for Perimenopausal Symptoms

Over half of all currently available prescriptions drugs are derived from plants. They are differentiated from the over-the-counter botanicals in that they have undergone rigorous trials for safety and efficacy and have been approved by the Food and Drug Administration. The 1994 Dietary Supplement Health and Education Act (DSHEA) made the Federal Trade Commission responsible for monitoring manufacturers of over-the-counter botanicals, now termed "dietary supplements." In 1997 the FDA ruled that the manufacturers of these supplements can promote claims of structural and functional improvement, but not disease treatment. Little regulation exists regarding the consistency of manufacture, quantity of active ingredients, safety, or shelf-life of these products.

Botanicals come in a variety of forms. Soy products are consumed in the form of beans, tofu, and soy milk. Whole herbs are sold dry in bulk at health food stores, as well as pulverized into tablet/caplet form, such as St. John's Wort tablets. Oils, such as flax seed and evening primrose, are concentrates of fat-soluble compounds. Tinctures are alcohol extracts and are often used in sublingual preparations. Teas, such as chamomile, extract the active ingredients by adding boiling water. The strength is determined by length of steeping time.

Teas, infusions, and decoctions are produced by increasing the length of steeping time. While the majority of botanicals are taken orally, some are manufactured as creams for transdermal use and in the form of enemas.

II. PHYTOESTROGENS

A. Biological Basis of Phytoestrogen Activities

Phytoestrogens are plant sterols that have varying affinities for human estrogen receptors. A variety of plant sources including soy, flax seed, red clover, and black cohosh are known to contain phytoestrogens. These supplements are used to treat perimenopausal symptoms perceived to be secondary to fluctuating or diminishing endogenous estrogen.

The three main classes of phytoestrogens are isoflavones, coumestans, and lignans. Isoflavones are the most common phytoestrogens and are found predominantly in leguminous plants, especially soy. Isoflavones have a diphesolic structure similar to diethylstilbestrol (6) (Fig. 1). The two major isoflavones, genistein and daidzein, are metabolized from their plant precursors biochenin A and formororetin, respectively. The content of isoflavones in various foods is shown in Table 2. Ipriflavone is a synthetic isoflavone derivative that is marketed as a food supplement.

Lignans occur in many plants as a minor component of the plant cell wall. They occur in whole grains, legumes, vegetables and seeds, with a high concentration in flax seed. Enterodactone and enterodiol are metabolites of the plant lignans matieresinol and secolsolariciresinol, respectively. Enterolactone and enterodiol are excreted in manmalian urine in proportion to the consumed precursors. Table 3 presents the lignan content of common foods (6).

Coumestrol is the major coumestan. It is found in high levels in the soy sprout as well as clover. It is found in smaller quantities in beans and peas (7,8).

Most American diets are fairly low in phytoestrogen content, with a daily genistein intake of 1 to 3 mg/day. In comparison, Asian populations consume 20 to 80 mg of genistein daily derived from soy. People who consume a vegetarian diet consume eightfold the amount of phytoestrogens as do omnivores (6).

Phytoestrogens are believed to exert their effects through binding to estrogen receptors. Because Asian populations report a lower frequency of menopausal symptoms and have a lower incidence of breast cancer, it has been proposed that phytoestrogens exert an agonist/antagonist effect on estrogen receptors. Compared to endogenous 17 β-estradiol, genistein has one-twentieth the binding affinity for estrogen receptor alpha (ER-α) and four-fifths the binding affinity for estrogen receptor beta (ER-β). Daidzein has a weak affinity for both receptors, and ipriflavone shows no binding activity. Coumestrol, however, binds equivalently to ER-β and has about one-third the binding activity of ER-α. Relative to estradiol, coumestrol and daidzein initiate the same amount of gene induction (activation) when bound to estrogen receptors, and genistein induced double the amount of activity (9). In vitro studies of phytoestrogens show a predominantly agonist effect at estrogen receptor sites. Genistein is an inhibitor of tyrosine protein kinase, DNA topoisomeres I and II, and ribosomal 56 kinase. Tyrosine kinases are active in tumorogenesis; inhibition of tyrosine kinase may be the source of genistein antiproliferative effect (10).

B. The Use of Isoflavones to Treat Perimenopausal Symptoms

Perimenopausal women increasingly use soy products to treat vasomotor symptoms and cycle irregularity. There is a growing body of evidence to support the efficacy of soy

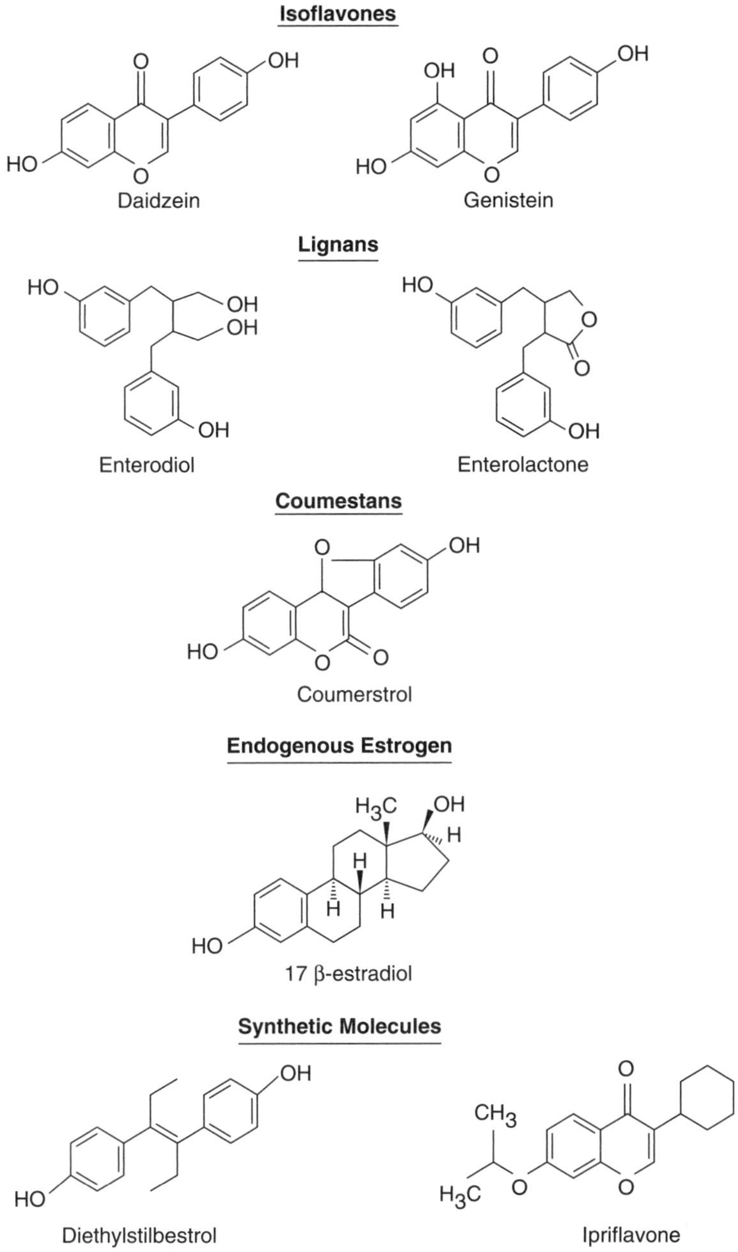

Isoflavones

Daidzein   Genistein

Lignans

Enterodiol   Enterolactone

Coumestans

Coumerstrol

Endogenous Estrogen

17 β-estradiol

Synthetic Molecules

Diethylstilbestrol   Ipriflavone

Figure 1 Structures of phytoestrogens and related compounds.

Table 2 Isoflavone Content in Food

Sources	Isoflavones (µg/g)
Soybeans	1800
Roasted soybeans	2600
Tofu (varies by brand)	300–500
Tempeh	865
Soy milk	450
Soy hot dogs	256
Soy sauce	150

Source: From Refs. 6,7.

Table 3 Lignan Content in Food

Sources	Lignans (μg/g)
Flax seed meal	675
Flax seed flour	526
Lentils	18
Wheat bran	5–7

Source: From Refs. 6,7.

isoflavones for the treatment of mild to moderate vasomotor symptoms. The data on cycle control is less convincing. Selected data are summarized in Table 4.

Muskies et al. in 1995 examined 58 postmenopausal women in a 12-week study comparing supplementation with 45 g of soy flour versus wheat flour on the effect of hot flashes. Compliance was measured by urinary daidzein levels. A 40% reduction in frequency and hot flashes was seen in the soy group, while a 25% reduction was noted in women in the wheat group (p < 0.001). The symptom relief occurred in the soy group earlier, within the first six weeks of the study. There was no significant change noted in vaginal cytology, FSH, or lipid profiles.

Albertazzi et al. performed a double-blind, multicenter trial to examine the effect of soy protein powder on the frequency of hot flashes in postmenopausal Italian women. Fifty-one women took 60 g of soy protein containing 76 mg of isoflavones (40 mg genistein, 28 mg daidzein, 8 mg others). Fifty-three women received 60 g of placebo containing no isoflavones. Women in the isoflavone group demonstrated reduction in hot

Table 4 Summary of Treatment of Hot Flashes with Isoflavones

Trial	Study design	Results
Murkies et al. (11) (II-1)	28 postmenopausal women given soy flour 30 postmenopausal women given wheat flour 12-week-controlled trial	40% reduction in hot flash frequency in soy 25% reduction in hot flash frequency in wheat
Albertazzi et al. (12) (II-1)	51 postmenopausal women given 76 mg isoflavones 53 placebo 12-week-placebo controlled trial	45% reduction in frequency of hot flashes in isoflavone group at 12 weeks 30% reduction on frequency in placebo
Baber et al. (12) (II-1)	51 postmenopausal women cross-over trial Postmenopausal women given 40 mg isoflavone or placebo	No statistical difference in vasomotor symptoms, but trend in improvement of 3x in active group
Van Patten et al. (15) (I)	59 breast cancer survivors received 90 mg isoflavones 65 breast cancer survivors received placebo Stratified for tamoxifen use for 12 weeks	Both groups had statistically significant decrease in hot flashes (i.e., strong placebo effect) No difference between groups
Jeri (16) (I)	15 postmenopausal women received Promensil (40 mg isoflavones) 15 women received placebo 16-week-trial	48% reduction in frequency of hot flashes in active group 10.5% reduction in frequency in control group

flashes of 26% at 3 weeks, 33% at 4 weeks, and 45% at 12 weeks, compared to a 40% reduction in the placebo group. Compliance and side effects were similar in each group (12).

Baber et al. studied supplementation of Promensil, a formulation containing 40 mg of isoflavones in a crossover trial of 51 women. Promensil is a commercially available preparation of red clover extract (13). The women were randomized to 12 weeks of active or placebo arms, with a one-month wash-out period between study arms. Although a trend toward decreased hot flashes was observed in the active arm, the difference was not statistically significant from placebo (14).

Van Patten et al. gave 90 mg of isoflavones versus placebo to Canadian breast cancer survivors. A statistically significant decrease in hot flashes was observed in both groups, but no differences were noted between the groups (15).

In another study of Promensil, 30 Peruvian women were randomized to receive treatment of placebo for 16 weeks. There was a 48% reduction in frequency of hot flashes in the Promensil group, versus 10.5% in the control group (p < 0.001).

Also noted in the treatment group was a statistically significant decrease in severity of hot flashes from 2.53 to 1.33, on a scale of 1 being light, 2 being moderate, and 3 being severe. FSH levels fell from 59 IU/ml to 48 IU/ml in the treatment group, and rose from 51 IU/ml to 54 IU/ml in the placebo group. These changes did not correlate to symptoms, and all levels remained in the postmenopausal range (16).

In summary, isoflavones reduce the frequency and severity of hot flashes in some women, although a strong placebo effect is seen in treatment of vasomotor symptoms (Level B). Unfortunately, all studies to date of treatment of vasomotor symptoms have been performed with postmenopausal patients. The etiology of hot flashes in perimenopausal patients is thought to be due to widely fluctuating levels of endogenous estrogen, as opposed to estrogen deficiency per se. Efficacy, therefore, of isoflavones used for treatment of hot flashes prior to menopause may differ from the experience in postmenopausal patients.

Menstrual irregularities are another common symptom of the perimenopause. Cassidy et al. studied the effect of adding 45 mg of isoflavones to the diet of six healthy premenopausal women with regular cycles. Women were monitored for one month prior to therapy, then received isoflavones daily for two months, then were monitored off the supplement. In five of six subjects, menstrual cycle length was increased by two to five days. Luteal phase length remained constant. Urinary levels of equol, a metabolite of diadzein and genistein, correlated with increasing follicular phase length. Midcycle levels of FSH and LH were suppressed when the women were taking isoflavones (II-2) (17).

In a follow-up study the same authors examined cycle length with doses of 25 g of isoflavones per day and noted a similar biologic effect (18). At this time there is insufficient data to recommend isoflavones for cycle control.

For women considering use of soy isoflavones to mitigate vasomotor symptoms, there exists reassuring safety data. Isoflavones have not been found to alter endometrial thickness or vaginal cytology (18,19). A study of ipriflavone, a synthetic isoflavone derivative, demonstrates an increase in bone density with doses of 600 mg/day. This increase was maintained after 24 months (20).

Many perimenopausal women are concerned about reducing their risk of breast cancer. Epidemiologic data suggests a lower incidence of breast cancer in Asian populations with a lifelong high intake of dietary phytoestrogens, especially soy isoflavores. Minimal data exists, however, on the safety of adding isoflavones in the perimenopausal years. In vitro studies of lignans on breast cancer cell lines have shown an inhibition of growth by 18% to 20% (10). Another in vitro study showed that low dose genistein stimulated growth of estrogen-sensitive breast cancer cells, while high dose genistein inhibited growth (21).

Petrakis et al. studied the effect of 38 mg of genistein taken daily on the lobular epithelium of the breast. Through nipple aspiration they found an increased secretion of breast fluid, the appearance of hyperplastic epithelial cells, and elevated levels of plasma estradiol in the premenopausal patients (22). This suggested a stimulatory effect, and caution should be advised regarding recommendation of isoflavones for reduction of breast cancer risk.

III. OTHER BOTANICALS USED FOR TREATMENT OF PERIMENOPAUSAL SYMPTOMS

A. Black cohosh *(Cimincifuga racemosa)*

Black cohosh, a perennial plant native to North America, has been used by Native Americans for treatment of menstrual problems. It has been approved by the German Commission E, which regulates herbal products, and has been used in Germany since the 1950s for the treatment of menopausal symptoms and dysmenorrhea. Remifenin is the brand name of the standardized extract, in tablet form, of the dried rhizone or root. The recommended dose, by the Commission E, is 40 mg/day (23). The key constituents of black cohosh are felt to be the triterpene glycosides, and the small level of the isoflavone formononetin, although the mechanism of action of black cohosh is unknown. Black cohosh contains small amounts of salicylic acid.

The NIH is currently funding research on black cohosh. A review of German studies demonstrated a significant reduction in menopausal symptoms through use of Remifenin; however, most of the trials were open, not placebo controlled (24). One double-blind German study did compare Remifenin with 0.625 mg of conjugated equine estrogen (CEE) and placebo. After eight weeks, Remifenin was found to have greater improvement in hot flashes, night sweats, and nervousness than placebo or CEE (25).

Black cohosh appears to be well tolerated. An overdose of black cohosh can cause nausea, vomiting, dizziness, or nervous system and visual disturbances. There are no known drug interactions (26). This needs a Level B recommendation.

B. Chasteberry *(Vitex Agnus Castus)*

Chasteberry, also known as Chaste Tree and Agnus Castus, is used for the treatment of PMS, fibroids, menstrual irregularities in the perimenopause, and breast pain. The extract, made from the dried ripe fruits of the Chaste tree, contains ingredients that inhibit prolactin through stimulation of D-type dopamine receptors (23). A randomized placebo-controlled trial of Chasteberry in groups of 50 women with breast pain demonstrated a reduction of premenstrual mastalgia (27).

A large randomized placebo-controlled trial has demonstrated improvement in PMS symptoms with use of Chasteberry. One hundred seventy women were randomized to receive a 20 mg tablet of standardized Chasteberry extract or placebo. PMS scores were taken before and at the end of three consecutive cycles. Significant improvement was seen in the treatment group for symptoms of irritability, mood alteration, headache, and breast fullness. Adverse effects were mild and there were no withdrawals from the treatment group (Level I) (28).

A German study of 52 women with luteal phase defects due to latent hyperprolactinemia demonstrated a normalization of luteal phase length and luteal phase progesterone after three months of therapy with Chasteberry extract (20 mg/day). The results were not seen in the placebo arm (II-1) (29).

Adverse reactions of chasteberry are rare and include itching, rash, alopecia, headaches, fatigue, agitation, tachycardia, and dry mouth (26). Drug interactions are unknown.

C. Dong quai *(Angelica sinensis)*

Dong quai, also known as Chinese angelica and Tang Kuei, is made from the root of Angelica sinensis. It has been prescribed in traditional Chinese medicine compounds for treatment of dysmenorrhea, irregular menstrual cycles, weakness during menses, and vasomotor symptoms. It is viewed as an adaptogen, restoring normal menstrual cyclicity. No randomized trials have been conducted evaluating the efficacy of Dong quai. Dong quai shows little estrogen receptor binding or estrogenic bioactivity (30). A number of case reports have documented potentialities of the effect of warfarin by Dong quai (31). Dong quai also can cause photosensitivity and photodermatitis.

D. Ginseng *(Panax ginseng, Panax quinquetolius)*

Ginseng is used in traditional Chinese medicine in order to increase estrogen for women at menopause. A trial in 584 women of ginseng versus placebo in Norway assessed quality of life, depression, and frequency of hot flashes by survey after 16 weeks of treatment. Also measured were FSH and estradiol levels, endometrial thickness, and vaginal cytology. A statistically significant improvement in depression was seen in the ginseng group. No difference was noted in vasomotor symptoms, hormone levels, endometrial thickness, or cytology (32).

Ginseng has been reported to potentiate the effects of caffeine. Side effects include insomnia, vaginal bleeding, Stevens Johnson syndrome, edema, hyperpyrexia, pruritus, hypotension, palpitations, headaches, and vertigo. Diarrhea and allergic reactions can occur with prolonged use or with large amounts of ginseng. Abuse has been reported (26).

E. Valerian Root *(Valerona officionalis L. valerianaceae)*

Perimenopausal women often report disordered sleep due to hot flashes. Valerian root has been used for centuries as a sedative. Its active ingredient is probably a gamma aminobutyne acid compound. No controlled trials were found regarding efficacy or safety, although adverse reactions such as headaches, excitability, and liver toxicity have been reported (33).

F. Other Botanicals Used for Perimenopausal Symptoms

The following (Table 5) lists other commonly used botanical agents for treatment of perimenopausal symptoms. No reliable trials have been found to confirm or deny efficacy or safety of these substances in the perimenopause or menopause.

Table 5 Other Agents Used for Perimenopausal Symptoms

Botanical	Purported Use	Caution
Kava kava	Treatment of anxiety	Possible addiction
St. John's Wort	Treatment of depression	Drug interaction; Photosensitivity
Damiona	Aphrodisiac	No known toxicity

IV. HOMEOPATHIC TREATMENTS OF PERIMENOPAUSAL SYMPTOMS

Homeopathy is a unique system of therapy based on the Law of Similars, which states that if a substance produces symptoms at high levels of ingestion, it can treat the same symptoms if ingested in minute quantities. Homeopathy is widely accepted in Europe and practiced by 20% to 30% of French and German physicians. Commonly used homeopathic agents are sepia for hot flashes, *calcarea carbonica* (carbonate of lime) for symptoms of heat, phosphorus and lachesis for vasomotor instability and sanguinaria (Blood Root) for flashing. None of these substances have been evaluated by clinical trials (26). One report of 20 postmenopausal women treated with the homeopathic medicine Feninon N noted a decrease in menopausal symptoms; however, the study was small and not controlled (34).

V. ACUPUNCTURE AND MASSAGE THERAPY

Classical acupuncture is a part of traditional Chinese medicine in which acupuncture needles are placed in specific anatomic locations and manually stimulated to treat many different health problems. In this therapy, acupuncture points, for example, Tai-xi Kl 3 between the medial malleolus and tendocalcaneous, are stimulated to relieve menopausal symptoms. No randomized controlled trials have studied the efficacy of acupuncture for treatment of menopausal symptoms. A small prospective study of 11 women who underwent acupuncture specifically for treatment of menopausal symptoms found nine women had significant improvement of vasomotor symptoms and fatigue that persisted for three months after termination of treatment. No change was noted in urinary incontinence or psychosexual function (35).

Massage therapy is used by both men and women to treat muscle strain and pain as well as to relieve anxiety and other stress-related symptoms. No trial has been published regarding efficacy of treatment for menopausal symptoms.

VI. CONCLUSIONS

Using the Evaluation System of the U.S. Preventive Services Task Force, use of isoflavones and Black Cohosh to treat hot flashes can be given B level of recommendation, with fair evidence from level I and II trials to support its use. Other botanical agents, homeopathy, acupuncture, and massage therapy await clinical trials to document safety and efficacy prior to recommending their use.

VII. RESOURCES FOR CLINICIANS

The following internet sites can be useful for patients and providers:

  i.   http://www.cfsan.fda.gov/~dms/supplmnt.html
       The Food and Drug Administration Center for Food Safety and Applied Nutrition's webpage about dietary supplements.
  ii. http://www.whccamp.hhs.gov/
       White House Commission on Complementary and Alternative Medicine Policy
  iii. http://nccam.nih.gov/

The National Center for Complementary and Alternative Medicine at the National Institutes of Health.

REFERENCES

1. Eisenberg DM, Davis RB, Ettner SL et al. Trends in alternative medicine use in the United States, 1990–1997. JAMA 1998; 280:1569–1575.
2. Newton KM, Buist DSM, Keenan NL et al. Use of alternative therapies for menopausal symptoms: results of a population-based survey. Obstet Gynecol 2002; 101(1):18–25.
3. Writing Group for the Women's Health Initiative Investigation. Risks and benefits of estrogen and progestin in healthy postmenopausal women. JAMA 1999; 288(3):321–333.
4. Studdert DM, Eisenberg MD, Miller FH et al. Medical malpractice implications of alternative medicine. JAMA 1998; 280(18):1610–1615.
5. InnoVision Communications. New model guidelines for the use of complementary and alternative therapies in medical practice. Int J Integrative Med 2002 Aug–Sept; 4(4):36–40.
6. Tham DM, Gardner CD, Haskell WL. Potential health benefits of dietary phytoestrogens: A review of the clinical, epidemiological and mechanistic evidence. J Clin Endocrinol Metab 1998; 83(7):2223–2238.
7. Bingham SA, Atkinson C, Liggins J et al. Phytoestrogens: Where are we now? Br J Nutrition 1998; 79:393–406.
8. Murkies AL, Wilcox G, Davis S. Phytoestrogens. J Clin Endocrinol Metab 1998; 83(2): 297–303.
9. Kuiper GGJM, Lemmen JG, Carlsson B et al. Interaction of estrogenic chemicals and phytoestrogens with estrogen receptor B. Endocrinology 1998; 139(10):4252–4263.
10. Knight DC, Eden JA. A review of the clinical effects of phytoestrogens. Obstet Gynecol 1996; 87:987–904.
11. Murkies AL, Lombard C, Strauss BJG et al. Dietary flour supplementation decreases postmenopausal hot flushes: Effect of soy and wheat. Maturitas 1995; pp 189–95.
12. Albertazzi P, Pansini F, Bonaccorsi G et al. The effect of dietary soy supplementation on hot flashes. Obstet Gynecol 1998; 91:6–11.
13. Fugh-Berman A, Krononberg F. Red clover (trifolium pratene) for menopausal women: Current state of knowledge. Menopause 1002; 1618(5):333–337.
14. Baber RJ, Templeman C, Morton T et al. Randomized placebo-controlled trial of an isoflavone supplement and menopausal symptoms in women. Climacteric 1999 June; 2(2):85–92.
15. Van Patten CL, Olivotto IA, Chambers GK et al. Effects of soy phytoestrogens on hot flashes in postmenopausal women with breast cancer: a randomized, controlled clinical trial. J Clin Oncol 2002; 20(6):1436–1438.
16. Jeri A. The use of an isoflavone supplement to relieve hot flushes. The Female Patient 2002; 27(1):35–37.
17. Cassidy A, Bingham S, Setchell K. Biological effects of a diet of soy protein rich in isoflavones on the menstrual cycle of perimenopausal women. Am J Clin Nutr 1994; 60:333–340.
18. Cassidy A, Bingham S, Setchell K. Biological effects of isoflavones in young women: importance of the chemical composition of soya bean products. Br J Nutr 1995; 74:587–601.
19. Murkies A. Phytoestrogens: What is the current knowledge? Aust Fam Phys 1998; 27(Suppl 1): 547–551.
20. Gambacciani M, Ciaponi M, Cappagli B et al. Effects of combined low dose of the isoflavone derivative ipriflavone and estrogen replacement on bone mineral density and metabolism in postmenopausal women. Maturitas 1997; 28:75–81.
21. Hudson T. Soy and women's health. Female Patient 2001; 26:26–34.
22. Petrakis NC, Barnes S, King EB et al. Stimulatory influence of soy protein isolate on breast sections in pre- and postmenopausal women. Cancer Epidemiol Biomarkers Prev 1996; 5(10):785–794.
23. Schulz V, Haensel R, Tyler VE. Rational phytotherapy: a physician's guide to herbal medicine. Berlin: Springer-Verlag 1998; pp 239–247.

24. Herbal medicine: Black cohosh: the woman's herb. Harvard Women's Health Watch 2000 April; 7(8):6.
25. Kass-Annese B. Alternative therapies for menopause. Clin Obstet Gynecol 2000; 43(1): 162–183.
26. Natural Medicine Comprehensive Database. Therapeutic Research Faculty. Stockton CA, 1999.
27. Halaste M, Raus K, Beles P et al. Treatment of cyclical mastadynia using an extract of Vitex agnus/castrus: results of a double-blind comparison with placebo. Ceska Gynekol 1998; 65(5): 388–392.
28. Schellenberg R. Treatment for the premenstrual syndrome with agnus castrus fruit extract: Prospective, randomized, placebo-controlled study. BMJ 2001; 322:132–137.
29. MilewiczA, Gejdel E, Sworen H et al. Vitex agnus castrus extract in the treatment of luteal phase defects due to latent hyperprolactinemia. Results of a randomized placebo-controlled double-blind study. Arzneimittelforwschung 1993; 43(7):752–756.
30. Zava DT, Dollbaum CM, Blen M. Estrogen and progestin bioactivity of foods, herbs, and spices. Proc Soc Exp Biol Med 1998; 217:369–378.
31. Page RL, Lawrence JD. Protentiation of warfarin by Dong quai. Pharmacotherapy 1999; 19(7):870–876.
32. Wiklund IK, Mattson LA, Lindgren R et al. Effects of standardized ginseng extract on quality of life and physiological parameters in symptomatic postmenopausal women: double-blind, placebo-controlled trial. Int J Clin Pharmacol Res 1999; 19(5):89–99.
33. Israel D, Youngkin EQ. Herbal therapies for perimenopausal and menopausal complaints. Pharmacotherapy 1997; 17(5):970–984.
34. Warenik-Szymankiewicz A, Meczekalski B, Obrebowska A. Feminon N in the treatment of menopausal symptoms. Ginekol Pol 1997; 68(2):89–93.
35. Dong H, Ludicke F, Comte I et al. An exploratory pilot study of acupuncture on the quality of life and reproductive hormone secretion of menopausal women. J Alternative Complementary Med 2001; 7(6):651–658.

2

Abnormal Uterine Bleeding During the Perimenopause

Alice S. Rhoton-Vlasak
Division of Reproductive Endocrinology and Infertility,
Department of Obstetrics and Gynecology, University of Florida College of Medicine,
Gainesville, Florida, U.S.A.

I. INTRODUCTION

Perimenopause has recently been defined at the stages of reproductive aging workshop (STRAW) held in July 2001. The perimenopause, which literally means "about or around the menopause," begins at the same time as the menopausal transition and ends one year after the final menstrual period. During this time, which is of variable length, menstrual cycles remain regular, but the duration changes by seven or more days, or may be characterized by two or more skipped menstrual periods and at least one intermenstrual interval of 60 days or more (1; Level III evidence). Thus, the perimenopause is characterized by increasing irregularity and unpredictability of menstrual cycles. Physiologic changes include an increasing incidence of short and long follicular phases, defective ovulation, anovulation, and highly erratic cycles. Often these changes are associated with premenstrual follicle stimulating hormone (FSH) elevations. The transition from ovulatory to luteal abnormality to anovulation is manifested clinically by intermenstrual lengthening and frequently menometrorrhagia. During this time, total estrogen levels are decreasing. Women frequently develop estrogen deficiency symptoms such as hot flashes, vaginal dryness, and frequency of urination, prior to having one year of amenorrhea.

Almost 90% of women will have four to eight years of menstrual cycle changes before menopause. It is important to distinguish irregular bleeding during the perimenopause from abnormal uterine bleeding. Abnormal uterine bleeding (AUB) in non-pregnant women is a common problem. It tends to be more common during the fifth decade of life (the perimenopausal years). AUB refers to the symptoms of excessive, prolonged, unexpected, or acyclic bleeding, regardless of diagnosis or cause, whereas dysfunctional uterine bleeding (DUB) is a diagnostic term for any abnormal bleeding from an essentially normal uterus. During the perimenopause, AUB is related to both aberrant hormonal function of the aging ovaries and to uterine abnormalities. This is reflected by the perimenopausal peak in hysterectomy rates for these indications (2). Various patterns of AUB are described in Table 1.

Table 1 Types of Abnormal Uterine Bleeding

Type	Bleeding pattern
Oligomenorrhea	Cycle length >35 days
Amenorrhea	Absence of bleeding for 3–6 months
Polymenorrhea	Cycle length <21 days
Menorrhagia	Excessive bleeding at regular intervals (>8 days, >80 ml)
Metrorrhagia	Irregular, frequent bleeding
Menometrorrhagia	Prolonged, excessive bleeding at irregular intervals
Intermenstrual bleeding	Bleeding that occurs between normal cycles
Hypomenorrhea	Cyclic bleeding with less flow than normal
Hypermenorrhea	Abnormal increase in the amount or duration of flow

The normal, non-pregnant, reproductive age woman ovulates every 21 to 35 days and in the absence of pregnancy has menstrual periods with the same interval. Menstrual periods usually last for 4 +/− 2 days, during which an average of 35 to 40 ml of blood is lost, an amount equivalent to 16 mg of iron. Whereas, the stated upper limit of normal is 80 ml, an amount that can be replaced by the recommended monthly dietary intake of iron, the average woman has been reported to become anemic if she loses more than 60 ml per month (3). Understanding the normal menstrual cycle duration is important in order to understand and recognize when bleeding becomes abnormal and requires further clinical evaluation. Our best information on menstrual cycle patterns during the perimenopausal transition comes from two longitudinal studies, the study of Vollman of more than 30,000 cycles recorded by 650 women and the study of Treloar of more than 25,000 women— years in slightly more than 27,000 women (4,5; Level II-3 evidence). Their data documented a normal evolution in length and variation of menstrual cycles. Vollman and Treloar noted increasing irregularity of cycles as menopause approaches, and specifically saw a sharp increase in cycle variability in 10% to 15% of women six years before menopause, which included increased numbers of short and long cycles. Also noted was a sharp increase in variability in another 30% of women between three and two years before menopause, although most women demonstrated little change in menstrual cycles until the last one to two years. Similarly, a chart review of 500 perimenopausal patients found that alterations in menstrual flow fit into one of three patterns: oligomenorrhea and/or hypomenorrhea (70%); menorrhagia, metrorrhagia, and/or hypermenorrhea (18%); and sudden amenorrhea (12%) (6; Level III evidence).

Although changes in bleeding pattern in perimenopausal patients are normal, it is critical for clinicians to recognize abnormal bleeding patterns so proper investigation can be undertaken. A recent study documented that more than two-third of gynecologic office visits by perimenopausal women were for AUB (7; Level III evidence). Unresolved AUB can have serious adverse consequences on a woman's health and on day-to-day living. Women can develop acute or chronic anemia, or find themselves at increased risk for pregnancy. Quality of life may diminish because of AUB, which interferes with activities of daily living, marital relationships, social interactions, and work. In the worst case, AUB may be a sign of atypical endometrial hyperplasia, which if undiagnosed and un-treated can progress to uterine cancer, the most common female genital cancer. Although uncommon among younger premenopausal women, the rate of endometrial neoplasia begins to increase sharply at age 45. Premalignant and malignant changes were present in 19% of perimenopausal patients with bleeding patterns other than amenorrhea or oligomenorrhea/hypomenorrhea (6). A careful menstrual history with particular attention to changes in menstrual patterns in perimenopausal women will help identify patients requiring further evaluation. The clinical management of patients with AUB or DUB is achieved with a combination of the following: history, physical examination, targeted use of laboratory evaluation, endometrial sampling, uterine imaging, and either medical or surgical therapy. This chapter will attempt to outline an evidence-based approach to the clinical management and treatment of AUB in perimenopausal women.

II. CAUSES OF ABNORMAL UTERINE BLEEDING

In the perimenopausal years, AUB is frequently related to DUB, which is either ovulatory or anovulatory. Dysfunctional uterine bleeding or anovulatory bleeding occurs during the reproductive years unrelated to structural uterine abnormalities. Ovulatory DUB occurs due to defects in local endometrial hemostasis; while anovulatory DUB is a systemic disorder, occurring due to the non-cyclic production of sex steroids in the absence of an anatomic lesion. Alternatively, abnormal bleeding may occur secondary to definable organic etiologies within the uterus that affect endometrial hemostasis, such as polyps, leiomyomas, and endometrial hyperplasia or neoplasia. Coagulopathies are uncommon but should at least be considered in the differential diagnosis of AUB. Table 2 outlines possible causes of AUB in perimenopausal women.

Uterine bleeding may occur in association with complications of pregnancy including abnormal and normal intrauterine gestation, ectopic pregnancy, and gestational trophoblastic disease. Abnormal intrauterine pregnancies comprise more than 50% of all gestations and are an extremely common cause of uterine bleeding. It is important to consider pregnancy related complications as a cause of bleeding in perimenopausal women since many of them have discontinued use of contraceptives as they no longer think they are at risk for pregnancy.

Table 2 Differential Diagnosis of Abnormal Uterine Bleeding in Perimenopausal Women

A.	**Organic causes**
	Benign reproductive tract disease
	Complications of pregnancy
	Leiomyomata uteri
	Polyps
	Adenomyosis
	Endometritis
	Cervicitis/vaginitis
	Premalignant/Malignant pelvic lesions
	Endometrial hyperplasia
	Endometrial adenocarcinoma
B.	**Systemic diseases**
	Coagulation disorders
	Hypothyroidism
	Liver disease
C.	**Iatrogenic causes**
	Hormone therapy
	Contraceptive devices/hormones
	Anticoagulation therapy
	Anovulation—Dysfunctional Uterine Bleeding

Source: Refs. 2, 8, 9.

Uterine leiomyomas are an extremely common finding, especially in women in the fourth and fifth decades of life. They are frequently associated with AUB, although many will present in asymptomatic women. Submucous myomas, involving the endometrial cavity usually cause menorrhagia due to interference with local hemostasis or expansion of the surface of the endometrial cavity. The clinician must remember that myomas that involve the endometrial cavity are often impossible to feel on manual examination. Consequently, the uterus normal to manual examination may indeed harbor a myoma that is causing the AUB. On the other hand, the myomas that are felt on clinical examination may not be the cause of bleeding experienced by the patient, particularly if they do not involve the endometrial cavity (10; Level III evidence). Figure 1 demonstrates an ultrasound image of an intramural uterine fibroid in a perimenopausal woman.

Endometrial or endocervical polyps are generally benign localized tumors that arise from either the endometrium or columnar epithelium of the cervix. Polyps may be visible on speculum exam, or only visible with imaging techniques or hysteroscopy (see Fig. 2). Polyps are generally not malignant and may be associated with a random bleeding pattern.

Adenomyosis is a benign condition characterized by the presence of endometrial glands and stroma within the myometrium. The gold standard for diagnosis is histological examination of a significant specimen of the myometrium at the time of hysterectomy. Women with adenomyosis most often present with menorrhagia, dysmenorrhea, and possibly an enlarged slightly "boggy" uterus on examination. Infections of the cervix or endometrium may also present with abnormal or post coital bleeding. Often a microorganism will be identified for treatment, or these infections may remain idiopathic. Endometritis may also occur following instrumentation of the uterus or pregnancy.

Although cancer is not the most common etiology of AUB in perimenopausal women, it is the most important to diagnose. Endometrial exposure to prolonged levels of unopposed estrogen stimulation, that frequently occurs with anovulation in the perimenopause may result in the development of endometrial hyperplasia. A study by Seltzer et al. in 1990 found that premalignant and malignant changes were present in 19% of perimenopausal patients with bleeding patterns other than amenorrhea or oligomenorrhea/hypermenorrhea (6; Level III evidence). Hyperplasia may be simple or complex and with or without atypia. Each entity places the patient at increased risk for endometrial cancer. Endometrial hyperplasia should be considered a cancer precursor, particularly when atypia is present (Table 3). A retrospective study of premenopausal women found that risk factors for endometrial

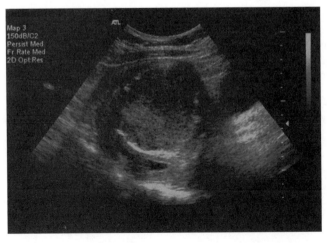

Figure 1 Transvaginal ultrasound image of an intramural leiomyoma impinging on the uterine cavity.

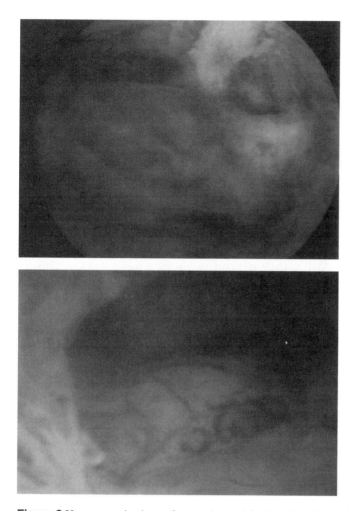

Figure 2 Hysteroscopic views of two endometrial polyps found in perimenopausal women with AUB.

hyperplasia in women with abnormal bleeding included body weight greater than 90 kg, age greater or equal to 45 years, infertility, family history of colonic carcinoma, and nulliparity. There was no increased association of endometrial hyperplasia on the basis of irregularity of the menstrual cycle, or the duration of menstrual bleeding (12; Level III evidence).

Women with congenital or acquired coagulopathies may present with AUB. Although these abnormalities are uncommon they are an important and often unrecognized cause of abnormal bleeding. Disorders of AUB may be related to platelet deficiency or

Table 3 Progression Rate of Untreated Endometrial Hyperplasia to Cancer

Type of hyperplasia*	Progression to cancer
Simple hyperplasia without atypia	1%
Complex hyperplasia without atypia	3%
Simple hyperplasia with atypia	8%
Complex hyperplasia with atypia	29%

Source: Ref. 11.
*Endometrial curettings obtained and patients followed for at least one year.

malfunction and/or prothrombin deficiency. Menorrhagia is a common symptom of von Willebrand's disease, which is a genetic condition characterized by a reduction in the quantity or quality of von Willebrand factor, a protein required for normal blood clotting. A recent prospective case control study of 121 women with menorrhagia (average age 35) found that bleeding disorders (von Willebrand's disease, factor deficiency, or platelet abnormality) were present in 10.7% of menorrhagic patients and 3.2% of controls (13). A separate analysis by race revealed a von Willebrand's disease prevalence of 15.9% among whites and 1.4% among black menorrhagic patients (14; Level II–2 evidence). Thrombocytopenia may result from a number of congenital and acquired conditions including bone marrow failure, cytotoxic drugs, hypersplenism, lymphoma, and a spectrum of metabolic diseases. Platelet numbers can be reduced by conditions that increase peripheral destruction, including non-immune causes such as vasculitis and thrombotic thrombocytopenic purpura, as well as more common immune etiologies such as autoimmune thrombocytopenic purpura (10).

Patients with hypothyroidism may present with AUB. It is important to check TSH levels in patients who present with menorrhagia. After replacement therapy is initiated, patients become euthyroid and AUB usually resolves within three to six months. Chronic liver disease and cirrhosis may be associated with excessive uterine bleeding due to reduced ability to metabolize estrogen and the inability of the liver to synthesize clotting factors. Severe liver disease causes levels of free estrogen to increase, causing endometrial hyperplasia and uterine bleeding (15). Iatrogenic causes of AUB include intrauterine devices and anticoagulants. More common causes would be oral, subdermal, or injectable steroids used for contraceptives, hormone replacement therapy, or other psychotropic medications.

Throughout the perimenopausal transition, there is a significant incidence of DUB due to anovulation. Dysfunctional uterine bleeding is diagnosed when abnormal bleeding occurs related to no demonstrable congenital or acquired causes. Both ovulatory and anovulatory DUB have been described. Ovulatory DUB is generally excessive bleeding associated with progesterone withdrawal, thereby manifesting predictable menses 21 to 35 days apart (10). Anovulatory DUB occurs in the absence of cyclic production of ovarian progesterone and, consequently is usually erratic in nature resulting in a mixture of amenorrhea and bleeding that is irregular in both timing and volume. Anemia is a frequent consequence of either type of DUB and in anovulatory DUB, the low levels of progesterone and exposure of the endometrium to elevated levels of estrogen facilitate the development of endometrial hyperplasia and endometrial adenocarcinoma (Figs. 3 and 4).

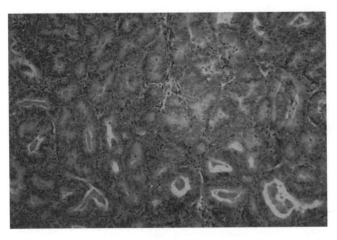

Figure 3 Histology views of well-differentiated endometrial adenocarcinoma.

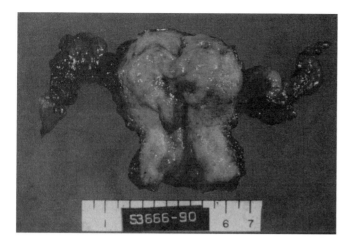

Figure 4 Surgical specimen showing endometrial adenocarcinoma with myometrial invasion.

III. CLINICAL INVESTIGATION

When a perimenopausal woman presents with AUB, the evaluation should begin with a careful history, physical examination, laboratory evaluation, and possibly imaging of the endometrial cavity. The clinician must learn to distinguish asymptomatic lesions from those that may contribute to bleeding problems. If the patient is hemodynamically stable, the history should detail the onset, frequency, duration of bleeding, cyclicity of bleeding, changes in previous menstrual patterns, and any associated pain. The history should determine to what extent the bleeding restricts daily activities. Other relevant factors in the history would include the sexual history, use of any contraceptives, other medications, detailed history of other systemic diseases, and possible symptoms of pregnancy.

Ovulatory status, is most cost effectively determined by history, as at least 95% of women with cyclic, predictable menses every 21 to 35 days are ovulatory (10; Level III evidence). Anovulatory bleeding patterns are typically irregular in timing and flow, and are often but not always interspersed with episodes of amenorrhea of varying duration. Also, relevant would be signs or symptoms of coagulopathy including easy bruising, family history of bleeding disorders, or bleeding with minor injuries. Weight gain or galactorrhea, marked fatigue, cold hands and feet, constipation, and failure to perspire in warm weather are potential signs of hypothyroidism.

A careful physical examination may offer further information on the cause of bleeding. Skin examination may reveal cold skin, that could be suggestive of hypothyroidism and signs of a coagulopathy such as petechiae. Breast examination may reveal evidence of galactorrhea. In a patient with a history of liver disease, careful abdominal exam should be done looking for evidence of jaundice, hepatomegaly, or ascites. Pelvic or lower abdominal pain, fever, and uterine or adnexal tenderness with a purulent cervical discharge suggest infection. Pelvic examination identifies severe infections, atrophy, cervical polyps, cervicitis, a prolapsed myoma, or even a lesion suspicious for cancer. An enlarged uterus suggests pregnancy, unless this has been ruled out, adenomyosis or possibly leiomyoma uteri.

Findings on physical examination that may suggest anovulation include obesity (BMI > 29) or extremely thin patients. Discrete disease entities known to cause anovulation may be suggested by hirsutism, thyromegaly, and galactorrhea. Acanthosis nigricans is frequently associated with insulin resistance and in combination with AUB is suggestive of polycystic ovary syndrome (16).

Diagnostic tests include a complete blood count, B-hCG, and cervical cytology. Select testing such as thyroid stimulating hormone (TSH), cervical cultures, coagulation parameters, and serum prolactin may be necessary in some cases depending on the outcome of the physical examination. For those women with associated mucous membrane bleeding (gums), epistaxis, bruising without petechiae, or a family history of abnormal bleeding, particularly with surgery or menses, von Willebrand's disease should be considered and factor VIII and ristocetin cofactor assays should be obtained (17). Gonadotropin levels are not useful in these situations since perimenopause represents a clinical diagnosis (1).

Clinicians should perform a rapid assessment to evaluate the patient's level of consciousness and stability of her vital signs. For unstable patients with profuse uterine bleeding, instant control can be achieved by placing a Foley catheter with a 30 ml balloon inside the uterus and inflating the balloon (15; Level III evidence). Immediate fluid resuscitation with crystalloid and blood are needed in severely anemic patients while deciding on the best treatment options.

A. Endometrial Evaluation

Comprehensive evaluation of abnormal bleeding in perimenopausal women in past years was primarily performed until the early 1980s by diagnostic dilatation and curettage (D&C) in the operating room under general anesthesia. However, endometrial evaluation has advanced to include endometrial sampling by office endometrial biopsy, visualization of the endometrial cavity by saline infusion sonography or hysteroscopy, and imaging of the uterus with ultrasound. These techniques can be used in a complementary fashion to evaluate and attempt to determine the cause of AUB.

B. Endometrial Biopsy

Office endometrial biopsy is one of the cornerstones in the diagnosis of endometrial pathology. The principal reason for obtaining endometrial histology in perimenopausal patients with AUB is to exclude the presence of endometrial hyperplasia or endometrial carcinoma. Prior to the development of flexible or rigid endometrial biopsy curettes, which have allowed the practice of endometrial biopsy to move into the office and become relatively inexpensive, diagnostic D&C in the operating room under general anesthesia remained the predominant method used to obtain samples. Now, a variety of sampling devices are available for office-based endometrial biopsy including reusable instruments (e.g., Novak and Vabra aspirator) and disposable devices (e.g., Pipelle and Tissue Trap). Numerous studies have shown that office endometrial biopsy using disposable or rigid catheters such as the Novak have been demonstrated equivalent to formal D&C (18, 19, 20; Level II evidence). Practitioners must remember that even D&C under general anesthesia may miss 2% to 6% of cases of cancer or hyperplasia (18–21). Current practice utilizes endometrial biopsies done with 3 to 4 mm sampling devices that usually do not require cervical dilation or anesthesia. A prospective randomized study comparing Pipelle endometrial sampling with the rigid Novak curette showed that Pipelle biopsy appears to be as effective as the Novak curette in obtaining an adequate specimen for histological analysis and is associated with less pain (22; Level I evidence). In patients with known endometrial carcinoma, a Pipelle endometrial biopsy prior to hysterectomy confirmed the diagnosis of endometrial carcinoma in 97.5% of patients yielding an extremely high sensitivity for the Pipelle endometrial sampling device (23; Level II evidence).

The technique of office endometrial biopsy is easy to learn and may be performed without assistance. Occasionally patients with cervical stenosis may require a formal D&C in the operating room. Endometrial biopsy is useful in the work-up of AUB in the peri-menopausal patient, cancer screening, endometrial dating, and infertility evaluation. Contraindications to the procedure include pregnancy, acute pelvic inflammatory disease, and acute cervical or vaginal infections. Cramping is the most common side effect and this is usually short-limited and mild. The rate of endometrial neoplasia begins to increase sharply at age 45 with up to 19% of women in one study showing premalignant and malignant changes on endometrial biopsy, so it is extremely important to utilize endometrial histology in diagnosing these patients (6). Since Pipelle endometrial biopsy samples a limited amount of endometrium, a patient having persistent symptoms despite a normal biopsy requires further evaluation. Office endometrial biopsy provides an adequate sample for assessing histology but is not useful for detecting anatomic abnormalities, so other methods are necessary to diagnose focal intrauterine lesions or other anatomic abnormalities.

C. Transvaginal Ultrasonography

Transvaginal ultrasonography (TVUS) of the pelvis is an important diagnostic procedure in the evaluation of perimenopausal women with AUB because it allows the detection of endometrial polyps or submucous fibroids, measurement of the endometrial thickness, and identification of ovarian masses. The procedure is a safe, inexpensive, and readily available technique to non-invasively image the uterus. An analysis of 35 studies enrolling more than 5000 women revealed that TVUS had a sensitivity of 96% in detecting cancer and 92.5% in detecting any proliferative abnormality in postmenopausal endometrium (upper limit of normal, 5 mm) (24; Level II evidence). A more recent study by Tabor et al. in symptomatic postmenopausal women reporting on the use of TVUS as compared to endometrial sampling in detecting endometrial cancer concluded that the measurement of endometrial thickness in symptomatic women does not reduce the need for invasive diagnostic testing, as 4% of cancers would have been missed, at a 50% false-positive rate. Furthermore, the authors noted statistically significant differences in endometrial thickness measurements between centers that studied the 4000 symptomatic women (25; Level II evidence).

Despite the wealth of data on evaluation of AUB in postmenopausal women, there is less information regarding ultrasonographic assessment of the premenopausal endometrium. Whereas a thin endometrium likely predicts the absence of endometrial hyperplasia or cancer, the physiologic impact of ovarian estrogens reduces the specificity of the test. A study of ultrasound-based triage for perimenopausal patients with AUB reported that unenhanced TVUS was sufficient for evaluating abnormal uterine bleeding in 65% of 433 women over the age of 39 who were not clinically menopausal (26; Level III evidence). If a thickened endometrial echo greater than 5 mm or no endometrial echo was reliably visualized, a saline infusion sonohysterography (SIS) was performed. 52% of 153 patients requiring SIS were found to have intrauterine polyps or myomas requiring hysteroscopic evaluation. Women with a symmetrically thickened endometrial stripe of greater than 3 mm in a single layer underwent office endometrial biopsy with histology detecting proliferative endometrium in 5, hyperplastic endo-metrium in 5. Figures 5A and B demonstrate TVUS images of normal and thickened endometrial echoes.

Saline infusion sonography (SIS) is extremely useful in determining the presence or absence of polyps or intracavitary leiomyomas that may contribute to AUB. It also provides

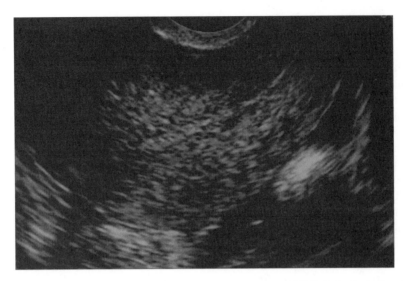

Figure 5A Transvaginal ultrasound image of a normal endometrial thickness.

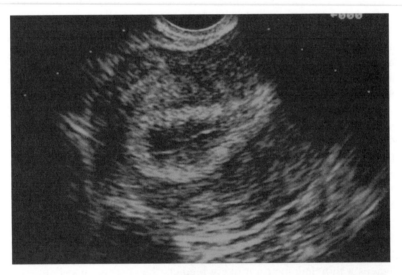

Figure 5B Transvaginal ultrasound image of a thickened endometrial stripe. (Figures 5A and B donated courtesy of Dr. Douglas Richards.)

information about the myometrium and its involvement with myomas not possible with hysteroscopic imaging. Figure 6 demonstrates a normal uterine cavity visualized by SIS. Saline infusion sonography has a sensitivity ranging from 99% to 100% for detecting intra-cavitary abnormalities in premenopausal women, therefore making SIS an extremely useful tool in the evaluation of perimenopausal women with abnormal uterine bleeding (27,28). Figures 7A and B demonstrate the usefulness of SIS to diagnose endometrial abnormalities not clearly seen with TVUS.

It is clear that TVUS and SIS are essential to the work-up of the patient with AUB, but using different cutoff levels for endometrial thickness with TVUS does not exclude polyps or hyperplasia in premenopausal patients, whereby TVUS should be combined with endometrial sampling and even hysteroscopy in selected premenopausal patients with

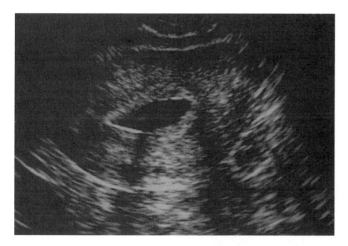

Figure 6 SIS demonstrating a normal uterine cavity and myometrium. (Figure donated courtesy of Dr. Douglas Richards.)

abnormal bleeding (29). The diagnostic accuracy of SIS is higher than the accuracy of TVUS. Dueholm found that SIS accurately identified all abnormalities except one, while TVUS alone left polyps undiagnosed in 20% of cases and resulted in equivocal findings in nearly 25% (28; Level II evidence). A combined approach of endometrial thickness by TVUS and reserving SIS for patients with increased (>5 mm) endometrial thickness, or endometrium inadequately visualized on TVUS, is the optimal method of reducing hysteroscopy rates (28).

D. Hysteroscopy

Until recently, hysteroscopy had been viewed as the gold standard for evaluating intracavitary lesions. Hysteroscopy is increasingly being replaced by SIS, a less invasive procedure that permits assessment of the myometrium and uterine cavity. The major disadvantage of SIS

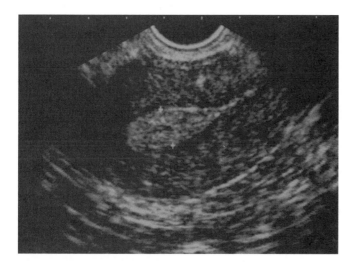

Figure 7A Transvaginal ultrasound image showing a thickened endometrium.

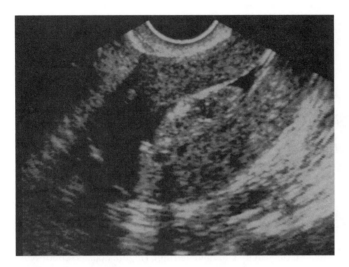

Figure 7B SIS on a patient from 8a demonstrating an endometrial polyp as the cause of the thickened endometrial stripe. (Figures donated courtesy of Dr. Douglas Richards.)

compared to hysteroscopy is the inability to obtain samples of lesions and other suspicious tissues. A recent prospective comparison of SIS with office hysteroscopy in 130 patients found that the sensitivity of SIS was 96% and specificity 88% compared with hysteroscopy, with the procedure of SIS being much less painful for patients (30; Level II evidence). A second prospective evaluation of sonohysterography in 233 pre- and postmenopausal patients with AUB found a sensitivity of 85.7% and a specificity of 95.4% in the diagnosis of polyps and submucous myomas (31). The evaluation of the endometrial cavity by office hysteroscopy and SIS, in studies of women with AUB, found a prevalence of polyps of between 24% and 41% and it was implied that polyps were the cause of the abnormal bleeding (32,33). A comparison of SIS findings in 100 asymptomatic premenopausal women age 30 and older and 80 premenopausal women of similar age with AUB found that those with abnormal bleeding had a higher prevalence of polyps (33 vs. 10%), intracavitary myomas (21 vs. 1%), and intramural myomas (58 vs. 13%) (34; Level II evidence).

If office hysteroscopy is available, diagnostic hysteroscopy can be performed in an office or clinic setting. Diagnostic hysteroscopy can be done quickly, safely, and with minimal discomfort. Unlike saline infusion sonography, it permits direct visualization of the endometrial cavity, identification of intracavitary lesions, and the possibility of removal and targeted biopsies. Office hysteroscopy also has the advantage of reducing costs. A U.S. cost analysis of hospital charges found costs were nearly 30 times those incurred when the procedure is performed in an office setting ($1799 vs. $64 U.S.) (35). Extreme discomfort in certain patients may preclude the use of office hysteroscopy, therefore requiring hysteroscopy under general anesthesia at a hospital or ambulatory surgery center. Diagnostic hysteroscopy has a very low complication rate. Review of 13,600 hysteroscopic procedures revealed a complication rate of 0.13% for diagnostic procedures and 0.28% for operative hysteroscopy (36; Level II evidence). Recent conflicting reports suggest that hysteroscopy may disseminate endometrial carcinoma cells—presumably the result of fluid insufflation, so it may be prudent to defer sonohysterography until office endometrial sampling has excluded carcinoma (8,37,38; Level III evidence).

There remains no reproducible and reliable way to diagnose adenomyosis. One study evaluated the usefulness of TVUS and uterine needle biopsy used singly or in combination in 102 premenopausal women scheduled for hysterectomy demonstrating a sensitivity of 82% for TVUS compared with 44% for uterine needle biopsy. Combining the

Table 4 Diagnostic Testing for AUB in Perimenopausal Women

History	
Physical examination	(Pap smear and cervical cultures)
Laboratory evaluation	Pregnancy test (B-hCG)
	Complete blood count (CBC)
	Thyroid stimulating hormone (TSH) Prolactin
Selected Patients	
	Coagulation studies
	Renal function tests
	Liver function tests
Other diagnostic testing	Office-based endometrial biopsy
	Transvaginal ultrasound
	Saline infusion sonogram
	Diagnostic hysteroscopy
After testing completed then triage to either medical or surgical therapy.	

tests did not improve the overall diagnostic performance for adenomyosis (39). A diagnostic or therapeutic D&C (in unstable patients) remains useful in women with cervical stenosis or other conditions that preclude SIS, office biopsy, or hysteroscopy. Practitioners may reserve hysteroscopy for women in whom intracavity lesions requiring biopsy or excision have been found by SIS (8). The diagnostic tests for evaluating patients with AUB in the perimenopausal women is outlined in Table 4. Approximate costs of various diagnostic tests and treatment options are listed in Table 5.

IV. TREATMENT OF ABNORMAL UTERINE BLEEDING

The treatment of AUB in the perimenopausal women depends on establishing the correct diagnosis. Medical rather than surgical therapy is the preferred management of AUB, especially if there is no associated pelvic pathology. There may be a specific therapy for coagulation disorders, hypothyroidism, and liver disease. If identified, iatrogenic causes should be eliminated. Treatment of anovulatory or dysfunctional uterine bleeding would begin initially with medical management to control bleeding and prevent the development of endometrial hyperplasia or endometrial cancer. Other specific etiologies such as uterine myomas, endometrial polyps, or adenomyosis may require surgical management including operative hysteroscopy, myomectomy, or hysterectomy.

Table 5 Costs of Diagnostic Testing Treatments Used in Perimenopausal Women with Abnormal Uterine Bleeding: Diagnostic Algorithm Costs

Procedure	Costs
History and physical examination	$150.00
Lab evaluation	$100–$200
Endometrial biopsy	$260.00
Transvaginal ultrasound	$270.00
Saline infusion sonogram	$311.00
Endometrial ablation	$4000.00
Operative hysteroscopy	$3575.00
Hysterectomy	$8000.00

The objectives and principles of treatment are to control the bleeding, prevent recurrences, potentially preserve fertility, and correct associated conditions. No single method is always effective so treatment may require attempting more than one method, possibly medical followed by surgical therapy if medical therapy is ineffective. In the triage for decisions regarding treatment of AUB therapy may depend on the acuteness of the bleeding episode. The first section of treatment options will review medical options for non-acute bleeding and the second section will review treatments for acute bleeding episodes. A common presenting symptom of women with AUB is fatigue secondary to anemia, which may be successfully treated with iron alone. It is important to initiate iron therapy in a daily dose of up to 60–180 mg of elemental iron as an essential component of any regimen for AUB.

Cyclooxygenase inhibitors (nonsteroidal antiinflammatory drugs—NSAIDS) such as diclofenac, flurbiprofen, ibuprofen, indomethacin, naproxen, and mefenamic acid have been evaluated in the treatment of AUB, especially in women with ovulatory DUB. Mefenamic acid and naproxen are typically prescribed in a dosage of 250 to 500 mg two to four times per day; ibuprofen has been studied in dosages ranging from 600 to 1200 mg per day. In a Cochrane review, five of seven randomized trials revealed that mean menstrual blood loss was less with NSAIDs than with placebo, and two showed no significant difference (40; Level I evidence). The review of the randomized controlled trials also revealed that NSAIDs are more effective than placebo, but are less effective than either tranexamic acid or Danazol. However, adverse events are more severe with Danazol therapy. In the limited number of small studies suitable for evaluation, no significant difference in efficacy was demonstrated between NSAIDs and other medical treatments such as oral luteal progesterone, antifibrinolytics, oral contraceptives, or progesterone intrauterine device (40; Level I evidence).

Antifibrinolytics are a mainstay of therapy for treatment of ovulatory menorrhagia in other parts of the world, but have rarely been used or studied in North America (41). An increase in levels of plasminogen activators have been found in the endometrium of women with AUB compared to those with normal menstrual blood loss. Plasminogen activator inhibitors (antifibrinolytic agents) have therefore been promoted as a treatment for heavy menstrual bleeding (42). There has been a reluctance to prescribe tranexamic acid due to possible side effects of the drugs such as an increased risk of deep venous thrombosis. Whereas small randomized controlled trials are not sufficient to exclude the possibility that such a relationship could exist, a retrospective study failed to show an association in a large cohort of women at enhanced risk for thromboembolic disease who were treated with tranexamic acid (43; Level III evidence). A Cochrane review in 2002 found seven randomized controlled trials of which four were available for review of antifibrinolytic therapy compared to placebo. The review showed a significant reduction in mean blood loss. Antifibrinolytic agents were compared to only three other medical therapies including mefenamic acid, norethisterone, and ethamsylate. In all instances there was a significant reduction in mean blood loss respectively with a strong, although non-significant trend in favor of tranexamic acid in the participants perception of an improvement in menstrual blood loss (42; Level I evidence). These studies did not reveal any associated increase in side effects compared to placebo, NSAIDs, oral luteal phase progestins, or ethamsylate. Unfortunately, the usefulness of antifibrinolytics is limited in the United States due to the fact that they are unavailable at this time.

Another frequently utilized option for medical management are hormonal methods including combination oral contraceptives, injectable monthly contraceptives, transdermal contraception, vaginal rings with a combination of estrogen, cyclic oral progestins, or continuous progestin (oral, injectable, or intrauterine device).

Estrogens plus progestins, in combination oral contraceptives or in lower hormone replacement doses, have been widely used in the treatment of AUB (Table 6). Today, a large

Table 6 Combination Estrogen/Progestin Therapies

Contraceptive formulations:

Cyclical

Low-dose (<35 µg ethinyl estradiol) combination oral contraceptives

Monthly contraceptive injection (medroxyprogesterone acetate 25 mg/estradiol cypionate 5 mg
  per injection)

Weekly transdermal contraceptive patch (150 µg norelgestromin/20 µg ethinyl estradiol daily)
  Three-week contraceptive vaginal ring (~120 µg etonogestrel/15 µg ethinyl estradiol per day)

Continuous

Three-month depot medroxyprogesterone acetate injection (150 mg per injection) plus oral or
  transdermal estrogen

Levonorgestrel intrauterine device plus estrogen

High progestin dose continuous combination menopausal formulations:

Norethindrone acetate 0.5 mg/estradiol 1 mg

Norethindrone acetate 1 mg/ethinyl estradiol 5 µg

Source: Ref. 8. Reprinted with permission from Contemporary OB/GYN and Dr. Andrew M. Kaunitz.

variety of estrogen/progestin options are available. Oral contraceptives are widely considered to be effective in the management of AUB occurring in otherwise healthy, non-smoking perimenopausal woman regardless of contraceptive needs (44). Despite their widespread use, only one published clinical trial has compared a monophasic oral contraceptive to mefenamic acid, naproxen, and low-dose Danazol in 45 women who were assigned to each of the four regimens for two months in an eight-month study, with oral contraceptives providing a reduction in bleeding that was similar to the other agents (45; Level I evidence).

An advantage of low-dose combination oral contraceptives is their relief of vasomotor symptoms, another common complaint in perimenopausal women. Oral contraceptives also make menstrual cycles more regular and decrease menstrual flow. A multicenter, randomized double-masked trial in over 200 women with AUB associated with anovulation treated with a triphasic norgestimate/35 µg ethinyl estradiol (EE) pill demonstrated improved bleeding patterns in 80% of subjects (46; Level I evidence). Another study over six cycles using an OC containing 20 µg EE/1 mg norethindrone acetate significantly shortened menstrual cycle duration, decreased variability, and reduced bleeding severity in 132 symptomatic perimenopausal women (47). Although the American College of Obstetricians and Gynecologists considers OCs the treatment of choice for anovulatory uterine bleeding, it is important to be aware that no combination estrogen-progestin formulation is FDA approved for the treatment of AUB in perimenopausal or other women (8; Level III evidence).

Because cycle control is an important issue for perimenopausal women who are experiencing AUB, the OC formulation selected should cause minimal breakthrough or irregular bleeding while minimizing the dose of EE. The rationale for minimizing the dose of EE is to maintain the lowest possible risk of a venous thrombo-embolism. Although three to four times higher than that of non-users, the risk of venous thrombo embolism (VTE) with newer low-dose OCs is substantially lower than that with the older higher dose OC's (48). Fortunately, this elevated risk does not appear to further increase with age (49). Oral contraceptives with 20 or 30 µg of EE are useful in the treatment of healthy non-smoking perimenopausal women with menorrhagia.

There is a group of perimenopausal women that will not be candidates for oral contraceptives due to cigarette smoking, hypertension, diabetes, or migraine headaches. In addition, women may have taken oral contraceptives in the past and are unable to tolerate them due to side effects such as nausea. Some clinicians choose not to use combination OCs in obese, perimenopausal women because combination OCs, advancing age, and obesity each represent independent VTE risk factors (49). Although progestins alone could be used in the group of high-risk women, those with vasomotor symptoms, low bone density, or hypoestrogenism associated with cigarette smoking may benefit more from an estrogen/progestin combination than from progestin alone (8). Options in women unable to take combination oral contraceptives include low-dose combined hormone replacement therapy or sequential estrogen progestin combination therapy. The main disadvantage is that often these regimens will not work well to control AUB. Continuous hormonal therapy combining progestin doses sufficient to suppress ovulation with doses of estrogen lower than those in combination OCs represents a useful therapeutic approach, although little if any data address this recommendation (8; Level III evidence). Two options reviewed by Kaunitz include a combination of oral or transdermal estradiol with depomedroxyprogesterone acetate injections, or the use of estradiol 1 mg plus norethindrone acetate 0.5 mg or EE 5 micrograms plus norethindrone acetate 1 mg daily. Each of these newer formulations provides endometrial suppression and good control of bleeding in late perimenopausal and postmenopausal women (50–53). Counsel perimenopausal women starting these new low estrogen, high progestin continuous combination regimens to initially expect irregular spotting/bleeding, with eventual bleeding patterns approaching amenorrhea (8).

Progestin-only options include oral progestin and the levonorgestrel intrauterine device (IUD). The major role of progestins is in the management of anovulatory DUB, which is a frequent cause of AUB in perimenopausal women. A variety of routes of administration and dosage schedules exist, ranging from intermittent luteal phase oral administration, through intramuscular injection, to continuous local administration by an IUD, each of which may have different efficacy in different clinical situations. North Americans almost invariably take medroxyprogesterone acetate (MPA), Provera for oral therapy but norethindrone acetate and norethindrone are also available. Table 7 lists suggested dosages, which should be administered for 12 to 14 days each month and usually result in predictable bleeding. Cyclic progestin therapy reverses hyperplastic changes in the majority of patients and controls irregular bleeding (54).

Despite the widespread and apparent usefulness of oral progestins in the management of AUB, there is little objective evidence to support their use, especially in women with ovulatory menorrhagia. A recent Cochrane review found seven randomized controlled trials for evaluation of which none compared progestin therapy with placebo. These studies showed progestins administered from day 15 or 19 to 26 of the cycle offered no advantage over other medical therapies such as Danazol, tranexamic acid, NSAIDs, and the progesterone releasing IUD for treatment of menorrhagia in women with ovulatory cycles.

Table 7 Oral Cyclic Progestin Therapy

Progestin	Tablet strengths (mg)	Daily dosage[a]
Medroxyprogesterone acetate (MPA)	2.5, 5.0, 10.0	5.0–10.0 mg
Norethindrone acetate	5.0	2.5–5.0 mg[b]
Norethindrone	0.35	0.7–1.0 mg[c]

[a]Administered for 12–14 days each month.
[b]1/2–1 Tablet/day.
[c]2–3 Tablets/day.
Source: Ref. 8. Reprinted with permission from Contemporary OB/GYN and Dr. Andrew M. Kaunitz.

Furthermore, progesterone therapy for 21 days of the cycle resulted in significant reductions in menstrual blood loss, although women found it less acceptable than the levonorgestrel IUD (55; Level I evidence). Progestins can be administered continuously in a dose of 10 to 20 mg per day of MPA or 5 mg per day of norethindrone, which usually results long-term in amenorrhea that is highly acceptable to many perimenopausal patients. Perimenopausal women whose endometrial biopsies show hyperplastic changes that do not wish to undergo hysterectomy could be placed on high-dose progestins for three months and re-biopsied to confirm reversal of hyperplasia.

The levonorgestrel releasing IUD is another treatment option for AUB. Many women find it desirable due to its usefulness to reduce menstrual bleeding, as well as the added benefit of offering highly effective contraception. Review of recently randomized controlled trials looking at the reduction in menstrual blood loss in women using the levonorgestrel IUD found that it was more effective than cyclic norethisterone (21 days) as a treatment for heavy menstrual bleeding (55; Level I evidence). The levonorgestrel IUD was also compared to transcervical resection of the endometrium and caused a smaller mean reduction in menstrual blood loss, but equal patient satisfaction with treatment. Interestingly, there is no data available from randomized controlled trials comparing the progesterone releasing IUD to either placebo, or other commonly used medical therapies for heavy menstrual bleeding (55). Among women awaiting hysterectomy, the planned surgery was canceled more often among those treated with the levonorgestrel IUD for six months, compared with those receiving their existing medical therapy (55). In a separate Finnish study that randomized women with menorrhagia referred for hysterectomy to either insertion of the levonorgestrel IUD or hysterectomy, patient satisfaction was similar in the two treatment groups at one year of follow-up (56; Level I evidence).

Kaunitz describes the insertion of a levonorgestrel IUD during the perimenopausal years, which can remain in place into the menopausal years with the addition of low-dose estrogen. This combination can relieve climacteric symptoms, maintain bone mineral density, and prevent genital atrophy while minimizing uterine bleeding and endometrial neoplasia (8; Level III evidence).

The androgenic steroid, Danazol, is effective for treating AUB. Daily doses of 200 or 400 mg were equally effective in reducing menstrual blood loss of more than 200 ml per pre-treatment cycle to less than 25 ml during a 12-week treatment phase (57). Although, effective in the control of AUB, Danazol is expensive and may have significant androgenic side effects such as weight gain, oily skin, and irreversible deepening of the voice.

GnRH agonist treatment results in medical menopause and creates amenorrhea. Despite the effectiveness of treatment in controlling bleeding, the menstrual blood loss returns after therapy is complete. Due to the expense and the side effects (hot flashes and osteoporosis) associated with GnRH agonists, the use of these agents in the long-term treatment of AUB is reserved for women with heavy blood loss who fail to respond to other methods of medical management and yet wish to avoid surgery. The use of addback estrogen and/or progestin therapy together with GnRH agonists will prevent the loss of bone associated with marked hypoestrogenism.

When leiomyomas are related to the bleeding, GnRH agonists frequently induce amenorrhea in association with shrinkage of both the myomas and total uterine volume. GnRH agonists may be useful in these situations to shrink myomas or reduce anemia prior to definitive surgical treatment with either myomectomy or hysterectomy. Most studies have demonstrated that myoma and uterine volume expand to pre-treatment levels within months of cessation of therapy (58,59; Level I evidence).

V. ACUTE UTERINE BLEEDING

Acute bleeding is controlled by estrogen, which promotes rapid regrowth of the endometrium over denuded epithelium. Oral conjugated equine estrogens (CEE), 10 mg a day in four divided doses (2.5 mg) may be used. Usually the bleeding is reduced within the first 24 hours after initiating treatment. Even after the bleeding stops, estrogen is continued for a total of 21 to 25 days and medroxyprogesterone acetate (MPA), 10 mg is administered concomitantly with the estrogen for the last 7 to 10 days. If the bleeding is not controlled within the first 48 hours, consider an organic cause.

Acute bleeding episodes can also be managed by CEE 25 mg administered intravenously every 2 to 4 hours for 24 hours. As with the oral administration of high-dose estrogen therapy, the amount of uterine bleeding is usually decreased within 24 hours. After the bleeding is controlled, oral CEE, 10 mg per day is prescribed for 21 to 25 days and then followed by oral CEE and MPA for another 7 to 10 days. A double-blind randomized controlled study in 34 patients to evaluate the efficacy of treating DUB with intravenous Premarin found that bleeding stopped in 72% of patients who received intravenous CEE and in 38% who received placebo (P = 0.021). Conjugated estrogen was effective in terminating endometrial bleeding in patients with biopsy proven pathology consisting of secretory, proliferative, menstrual, polyploid, or cystic hyperplasia, as well as endometritis (60; Level I evidence).

Another treatment of acute bleeding in non-smokers is a combination oral contraceptive, three to four tablets per day. After the bleeding stops treatment is continued for at least one more week. Progestins alone usually are not effective in stopping an acute bleeding episode, but are indicated for the long-term treatment once the acute bleeding episode has resolved (15) (Table 8).

VI. SURGICAL MANAGEMENT OF ABNORMAL UTERINE BLEEDING

If bleeding continues despite medical therapy, surgical intervention is indicated. Surgical treatment such as operative hysteroscopy, myomectomy, or hysterectomy is indicated in women found to have endometrial polyps, uterine leiomyomas, endometrial hyperplasia, or carcinoma. Hysterectomy is no longer considered to be the only definitive cure for patients with benign AUB. Approximately 600,000 hysterectomies are performed annually in the United States, making this the second most frequently performed major surgical

Table 8 Treatment Options for Acute Bleeding[a]

1.	Conjugated equine estrogen (CEE) IV every 4 hours until bleeding stops or for 24 hours followed by oral CEE[b] 10 mg for 28 days. Add medroxyprogesterone acetate (MPA) 10 mg daily for the last 10 days.
	OR
2.	Oral CEE[b] 2.5 mg po qid × 24 hours, then oral CEE 10 mg × 21–25 days. Add MPA 10 mg daily for the last 7 days.
	OR
3.	(In non-smokers) Low-dose monophasic oral contraceptive 2–4 times daily for one week, followed by one pill daily.

[a]If bleeding is not controlled within 24–48 hours, consider an organic cause or surgical intervention.
[b]CEE: Conjugated equine estrogen.
Sources: Refs. 15, 60.

procedure among reproductive aged women (61,62). Among women age 35 to 54, the diagnosis most often associated with hysterectomy is uterine leiomyoma. Seventy-six percent of women age 45 to 54 undergoing hysterectomy had a concomitant oophorectomy (61).

A D&C can be both diagnostic and therapeutic for patients with menorrhagia who are hypovolemic or unstable from acute bleeding. Dilation and curettage is otherwise considered obsolete for the evaluation and treatment of AUB because it is inaccurate, does not detect intracavity lesions, and 60% of patients will develop a recurrence of AUB. Therefore, if a patient has a curettage revealing histologic evidence of anovulatory bleeding, they should receive MPA each month as previously described (15).

Traditionally, D&C was used to diagnose the cause of excessive uterine bleeding in patients older than 35 years, when the incidence of neoplastic lesions increase or when the patient has endometrial hyperplasia as determined by endometrial biopsy. Hysteroscopic examination of the endometrial cavity is superior to D&C because it allows direct visualization of the endometrial cavity, identification of polyps and submucous myomas, as well as directed biopsies of the most suspicious areas (8). Histological specimens should always be sent from any invasive procedures on perimenopausal women with AUB in order to rule out the presence of a malignancy. (Fig. 3).

Operative hysteroscopy has increasingly been used to treat women with intrauterine pathology such as polyps or submucous myomas, or as a means to perform endometrial ablation. Several studies have looked at the usefulness of hysteroscopic myomectomy and found that this gives satisfactory control of menorrhagia with a limited chance for recurrence (63,64). Vercellini studied 108 women who had first line hysteroscopic resection of submucous myomas. He found myomas recurred in 34% with a probability of three-year recurrence of menorrhagia of 30%. Also, myoma intramural extension did not have a substantial influence on any of the long-term outcomes, but affected operating time and the number of procedures needed for complete removal (63). Endometrial polyps are also amenable to removal by operative hysteroscopy usually resulting in a short, relatively safe outpatient procedure. Figures 8A and 8B demonstrate SIS pictures of a submucous myoma and hysteroscopic view prior to complete hysteroscopic resection.

Hysteroscopic endometrial resection and ablation are very useful in menorrhagic patients who wish to avoid hysterectomy.

A. Endometrial Ablation

Endometrial ablation is a surgical technique that selectively destroys the endometrium. Hysteroscopically directed endometrial ablation was introduced as an alternative to hysterectomy for menorrhagic women at high surgical risk because of significant co-existent medical conditions (65). Endometrial ablation is most useful in women with no anatomic uterine pathology such as leiomyoma, patients refusing hysterectomy with AUB, or poor surgical candidates. The procedure is more successful in treating women in their 40s compared with women in their 30s. (66,67; Level II evidence) Boujida et al. found that younger women were much more likely to require second ablation or hysterectomy compared to older women (67). Perimenopausal patients with endometrial hyperplasia or neoplasia are not candidates for endometrial ablation, but require definitive surgical treatment and referral to a gynecologic oncologist. Endometrial ablation has the advantages of a short hospital stay, absence of surgical incisions, and subsequent rapid return to normal activity. All endometrial ablation procedures should be preceded by endometrial sampling to rule out the presence of endometrial hyperplasia or neoplasia prior to the surgical procedure.

One of the main problems of endometrial ablation is evaluating the uterine cavity adequately in the menopause if uterine bleeding occurs on or off hormone replacement therapy.

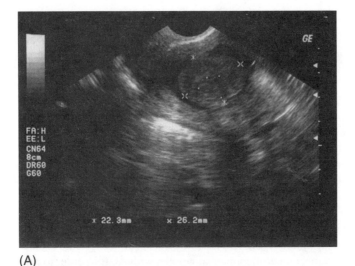

(A)

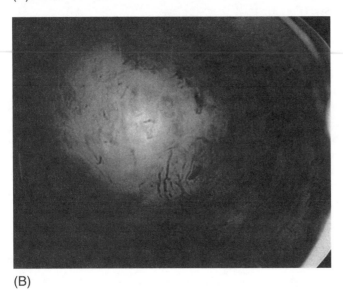

(B)

Figure 8 (A) SIS demonstrating a 2-cm submucous myoma in a woman with menorrhagia. (B) Hysteroscopic view of 2-cm submucous myoma just prior to resection.

Women with ablated endometrial cavities may have difficulty undergoing office endometrial biopsies. Even in the operating room with a hysteroscope, the scarring makes evaluating the cavity somewhat difficult. Therefore, in perimenopausal women in whom menorrhagia has persisted despite medical therapy and who have completed their families, hysterectomy remains a therapy of choice. Several options exist for endometrial ablation. The original techniques designed were hysteroscopically directed methods for resection or destruction of the endometrium. However, it has been recognized that optimal outcomes with hysteroscopic endometrial ablation require a level of skill and experience that may not be achieved by the average surgeon (68).

Potential advantages of endometrial resection or resection/ablation include histologic sampling of the endometrium, lower risk of subsequently concealed endometrial hyperplasia or carcinoma, and reduced need for preoperative hormonal preparation of the endometrium.

Unanticipated submucous myomas or polyps can be simultaneously resected without need to change instrumentation or to discontinue the procedure (68). The disadvantages of hysteroscopic techniques include the requirement for better hysteroscopic skills and more extensive understanding of the uterine anatomy. Complications of hysteroscopic endometrial ablation include anesthesia complications, uterine perforation, infection, hemorrhage, and systemic absorption of distension media causing hyponatremia or hyposmolarity. A recent Cochrane Review (Class I evidence) of endometrial resection and ablation versus hysterectomy for heavy menstrual bleeding found there was a significant advantage in favor of hysterectomy in the improvement of heavy menstrual bleeding and satisfaction rates compared with endometrial destruction techniques (69). Duration of surgery, hospital stay, and recovery time were all shorter following endometrial destruction. The total cost of endometrial destruction was significantly lower than the cost of hysterectomy, but the difference between the two procedures narrowed over time because of the high cost of retreatment in the endometrial destruction group (69).

Hysteroscopic endometrial ablation can be accomplished with several means including laser, electrical, or thermal energy, or resection with a loop electrode deployed by a modified urologic resectoscope. A series of 401 patients who underwent endometrial ablation with laser hysteroscopic endometrial ablation with the Nd:YAG laser versus electrosurgical resection were followed for a minimum of one year with amenorrhea developing in 58% of patients, 34% with light or normal menstrual flow, and 8% did not respond and had continued heavy flow (70). The study demonstrated that hysteroscopic endometrial ablation is a reliable, safe alternative to hysterectomy for the surgical management of AUB (70; Level III evidence). A randomized prospective study of premenopausal menorrhagic women with normal hysteroscopic and endometrial biopsy findings randomly assigned patients to endometrial vaporization, or endometrial resection with follow-up menstrual pattern evaluation at one year revealed a 100% improvement in bleeding in the endometrial vaporization group and 96% improvement in the endometrial resection group (71; Level II evidence). Endometrial ablation with the vaporizing electrode limited fluid absorption compared with resection by the standard cutting loop.

As an alternative to the hysteroscopic endometrial ablation, non-hysteroscopic endometrial ablation techniques were developed. Treatments for menorrhagia by blind destruction of the endometrium require less surgical skill and minimize the risk of fluid overload from the absorption of uterine distension media. A variety of methods have been proposed or demonstrated including electrosurgical techniques, cryotherapy, microwave, hyperthermia, diode lasers, and photosensitizers (68). The simplest non-hysteroscopic endometrial ablation technique is the thermal balloon (ThermaChoice uterine balloon therapy system), which is filled with a solution of sterile dextrose and water and then heated to 87°C for eight minutes. In a multicenter randomized controlled trial, Meyer and colleagues demonstrated that at 12 and 24 months outcome of surgical balloon therapy was equivalent to roller ball desiccation in terms of bleeding response and patient satisfaction (72,73; Level I evidence). Bongers et al. in 2002 found a cumulative hysterectomy rate within two years after a thermal ablation of 12% with 81% of patients still satisfied with the treatment (74). Young age, retroverted uterus, endometrial thickness more than 4 mm, and a prolonged duration of menstruation were associated with an increased rate of treatment failure (74). The thermal balloon limits uterine size to a sounded length of 10 cm.

A newer technique for endometrial ablation uses saline heated to 90°C and circulated in the uterine cavity for 10 minutes under hysteroscopic control (75). Corson found in a randomized prospective multicenter trial that success rates in women treated for menorrhagia due to benign causes were 77% for the heated saline technique and 82% for endometrial roller ball endometrial ablation (76; Level I evidence). Advantages of the heated saline technique include its office-based nature, reduction of the requirement for anesthesia, and obviating the problems of fluid absorption (8). Other options for non-hysteroscopic endometrial ablation include a bipolar electrode, microwave energy, and photodynamic therapy (68). A Scottish randomized trial of ablation by microwave versus endometrial resection (with two years of follow-up) demonstrated a 79% versus 67% satisfaction rate, similar hysterectomy rates (11 vs. 12%), and similar menstrual improvement (77; Level I evidence). The average amenorrhea rate ranges from 20% to 40% (72–77). Around 90% of women experience a satisfactory reduction in menstrual bleeding.

High quality evidence from a Cochrane Review (Class I Evidence) supports the use of GnRH agonists pretreatment for endometrial ablation. Pretreatment with GnRH agonists was associated with a shorter duration of surgery, greater ease of surgery, and a higher rate of postoperative amenorrhea. GnRH agonists produced more consistent endometrial atrophy than Danazol and limited randomized data was available to assess the effectiveness of progestins as endometrial thinning agents (78).

B. Hysterectomy

Definitive treatment of patients with AUB failing medical treatment or conservative surgery remains hysterectomy, but this is a major surgical procedure with significant physical and emotional complications as well as social and economic costs. Of the half-million hysterectomies performed every year in the United States, 50% or more are for treatment of abnormal uterine bleeding (41). Patients need to be counseled carefully prior to the surgery regarding the surgical risks, the fact that surgery will eliminate their fertility, and to discuss whether oophorectomy should be performed. The most recent review of randomized comparisons of hysterectomy with endometrial destruction techniques for treatment of heavy menstrual bleeding in premenopausal women analyzed five trials (69).

The review found a significant advantage in favor of hysterectomy in the improvement of menorrhagia and satisfaction rates up to four years post surgery compared with endometrial destruction techniques (69; Level I evidence). Although hysterectomy is associated with a longer operating time, a longer recovery period, and higher rates of postoperative complications, it offers permanent relief from heavy menstrual bleeding. In randomized trials of hysterectomy and endometrial ablation, women after hysterectomy have better quality of life and higher levels of satisfaction with treatment than women after endometrial ablation (79). A review of 497 women undergoing hysterectomies between 1993 and 1995 revealed that the most common indications for hysterectomy were leiomyomata (60%), pelvic relaxation (11%), pain (9%), and bleeding (8%). Of the hysterectomies, 367 (70%) did not meet the level of care recommended by the expert panel and were judged to be recommended inappropriately (80). Thus, patients and physicians should work together to ensure that proper diagnostic evaluation has been done and appropriate treatments considered before hysterectomy is recommended.

Structural pathologies of the uterus known to be associated with AUB include leiomyomas, polyps, adenomyosis, and endometrial hyperplasia or neoplasia. It is important to remember that benign processes may be entirely asymptomatic, making clinical correlation a necessary component of the investigative process (10). Perimenopausal women found to have endometrial polyps as the cause of AUB have the option of hysteroscopic resection or hysterectomy. Endometrial neoplasia or hyperplasia usually necessitates surgical treatment and possible evaluation by a gynecologic oncologist.

Perimenopausal women with AUB found to have uterine fibroids now have several options for treatment including conservative uterine retaining surgery with an abdominal myomectomy, hysterectomy, or uterine artery embolization. There is high quality evidence that preoperative administration of GnRH agonists is beneficial pre-myomectomy in selected patients (81; Level I evidence). In anemic women, creation of amenorrhea can be expected to facilitate restoration of hemoglobin levels, provided sufficient amounts of iron are administered over an adequate amount of time.

C. Minimally Invasive Surgical Management

Newer techniques such as laparoscopic myomectomy and cryotherapy or "myolysis" are being used selectively at a limited number of centers where these techniques are available. Stovall et al. performed a randomized trial of women with 14- to 18- week-size uterus randomized into two groups to determine whether preoperative GnRH agonists would increase the feasibility of vaginal rather than abdominal hysterectomy. Patients treated with GnRH agonists were more likely to have increased hemoglobin levels and decreased uterine volume after eight weeks of agonist therapy and were more likely to undergo vaginal hysterectomy, allowing a significantly shorter hospital stay (82; Level I evidence). Another experimental technique available for women with uterine leiomyomas who desire neither hysterectomy nor further child bearing is uterine artery embolization. The patient undergoes a combination of local anesthesia with conscious sedation and analgesia. A radiologist catheterizes one femoral artery and under fluoroscopic guidance manipulates the catheter in a retrograde fashion up the femoral, then through the external and internal iliac arteries and positions the tip in the uterine artery, where polyvinyl alcohol particles embolize the vessels. The patient may experience a significant amount of pain in the first 24 hours, therefore frequently requiring hospital admission for parenteral analgesia. Available clinical data consists mostly of case series. Myoma shrinkage averages approximately 50% to 70%, and patients with AUB experience control of symptoms at least 85% of the time and in one series 100% at one year (83,84; Level III evidence). Patients must be counseled that uterine artery embolization is a procedure in development, that its impact on any future pregnancies is at best unknown and at worst could be disastrous if the patient requires an emergency hysterectomy following the procedure. The decision should be individualized after discussion and collaboration among gynecologists, interventional radiologists, and other relevant health care providers (68).

Adenomyosis may be associated with dysmenorrhea and AUB in perimenopausal patients and continues to constitute a common indication for hysterectomy and is often encountered on pathological examination of the uterus. It remains difficult to diagnose preoperatively and even attempts at transvaginal ultrasound-guided biopsy have limited diagnostic usefulness (39).

Surgical management of AUB is in a process of evolution, from one in which hysterectomy was the only choice, to one in which there exists a multitude of approaches, each of which has different risks, costs, clinical outcomes, and appropriateness for a given patient. It is important to be aware of these options and to present these to perimenopausal women presenting with AUB so they can choose a surgery that best fits their reproductive desires, as well as adequately address their bleeding. In addition, non-surgical techniques ranging from uterine artery embolization through newly packaged devices such as progesterone-containing IUDs may each find a particular niche in the management of appropriately selected women with AUB.

VII. ALTERNATIVE MEDICINES

Despite the multitude of traditional evidenced-based medical and surgical therapies available for treatment of perimenopausal women with AUB, and due to the perceived benefits of herbal medicines, many women are turning to these for treatment. Women are looking for hormone therapy to treat vasomotor symptoms, possible premenstrual syndrome, dysmenorrhea, and complaints of menstrual disorders that are very common in perimenopausal women. At this time, approximately one-third of North Americans older than 18 years of age use herbal remedies for numerous illnesses; 53% are convinced of their therapeutic efficacy, and 65% of their safety (85). Many suggested alternative therapies include lifestyle changes, vitamins, dietary changes, and other remedies that do not require a Z prescription. It is most important for patients to understand that herbs are drugs. Patients must also understand that even though herbal medicines are sold in places such as health food stores and grocery stores that they may not be always safe.

Phytoestrogens are naturally occurring compounds found in many foods, consisting of a number of classes that include lignans, isoflavones, coumestans, and resorcylic acid lactones. The isoflavones are generally restricted to legumes, with the highest concentrations found in soy beans and soy products. Lignans are found in almost all cereals and vegetables with the highest concentration in the oil seeds, especially linseed and flax seed (86). Phytoestrogens have been most commonly used as a means to alleviate hot flashes. There is no evidence that increased dietary intake of these products increases the risk of cancer. In Asia and Eastern Europe, where these products are consumed more than in Western nations, the incidence of breast, colon, endometrial, and ovarian cancer are all lower (87; Level III evidence). Dietary phytoestrogens may result in unopposed estrogen activity in low estrogen states or after menopause. No data is available concerning endometrial growth secondary to high dietary phytoestrogens. However, as stated above, there is no increased incidence in endometrial cancer reported from countries with high intake levels of phytoestrogens (88).

A recent review in pharmacotherapy on herbal therapies for perimenopausal and menopausal women suggested that four herbs have usefulness in menstrual irregularities: Angelica, Chasteberry (*Vitex Agnus-Castus*), Dandelion (*Taraxacum officinale*), and Fenugreek (*Trigonella foenum-Graecum*) (89; Level III evidence). Despite the claims for any of these herbal therapies, there is no good scientific evidence to support their use in treatment of menstrual disorders in perimenopausal women. Other herbal therapies available for treatment of perimenopausal vasomotor symptoms are discussed in the chapter on the use of herbal medicines in perimenopausal patients. Chinese medical and herbal practitioners frequently practice acupuncture as treatment for a variety of different disorders. A series of 50 cases of women with dysfunctional uterine bleeding both ovulatory and anovulatory were treated effectively with acupuncture (90).

Most importantly, practitioners should remember that patients will frequently take herbs that they may or may not report in review of their medications. Since a number of herbs have been associated with potentially increased bleeding, it is important to obtain this information in the history of any perimenopausal patient presenting with AUB. Recently recognized herbal medicines associated with potential increased bleeding include garlic, feverview, ginger, ginseng, and gingko biloba (91,92). It is vital for physicians to be apprised of all substances ingested by patients, to be cognizant of their potential adverse effects and drug interactions, and to be familiar with their therapeutic modalities, all of which help to optimize therapeutic approaches and improve patient outcome.

VIII. SUMMARY

A hallmark of the perimenopausal transition is AUB. In perimenopausal women with normal findings on physical examination, the most likely diagnosis is dysfunctional uterine bleeding secondary to anovulation. Since other etiologies increase in prevalence in perimenopausal patients, it is important to undertake a careful history and physical exam, as well as diagnostic testing to complete the investigation. In perimenopausal patients, endometrial biopsy, transvaginal ultrasound, and saline infusion sonogram are very useful in detecting endometrial pathology. Diagnostic hysteroscopy is utilized for recalcitrant bleeding, or in an office-based setting if this is available. Once a diagnosis for the bleeding has been determined and neoplasia has been ruled out, there are several variables that should be considered in deciding on the treatment course including the patient's need for contraception, contraindications to estrogen, and pathology on endometrial biopsy.

Initial management would usually consist of hormonal treatment with either low-dose estrogen progestin contraceptives, or progestins. Patients with adenomatous hyperplasia with no or mild atypia may be treated with high-dose medroxyprogesterone acetate for several months and then re-biopsied. Patients with moderate or severe atypia should be encouraged to have a hysterectomy. Surgical management options are directed by the type of uterine pathology, which is identified in patients. Patients with dysfunctional bleeding in which no organic pathology is found and fails to respond to medical therapy are candidates for either endometrial ablation procedures, or vaginal or abdominal hysterectomy. The decision to retain the ovaries or not should be carefully discussed with the patient and be decided prior to the surgical procedures. Perimenopausal patients who choose to undergo treatment with hysterectomy and bilateral salpingo-oophorectomy should be counseled on the recommendation for estrogen replacement therapy prior to surgery. With careful diagnostic evaluation and stepwise treatment, clinicians are able to improve perimenopausal women's quality of life and deal with AUB that is very common during this transitional period. It is also important in perimenopausal women always to consider the possibility of pregnancy as a cause of bleeding and rule this out early on in the evaluation.

REFERENCES

1. Soules MR, Sherman S, Parrott E et al. Executive summary: Stages of reproductive aging workshop (STRAW). Fertil Steril 2001; 76:874–878.
2. Wilcox LS, Koonin LM, Pokras R et al. Hysterectomy in the United States, 1988–1990. Obstet Gynecol 1994; 83:549–555.
3. Hallberg L, Hogdahl A, Nilsson L et al. Menstrual blood loss—A population study. Acta Obstet Gynecol Scand 1996; 45:320–351.
4. Vollman RF. The menstrual cycle. Major problems in Obstetrics and Gynecology. Philadelphia, PA: W.B. Saunders Company, 1977.
5. Treloar AE, Boynton RE, Behn BG et al. Variation of the human menstrual cycle through reproductive life. Int J Fertil 1970; 12:7–126.
6. Seltzer VL, Benjamin F, Deutsch S. Perimenopausal bleeding patterns and pathologic findings. J Am Med Womens Assoc 1990; 45:132–134.
7. Mencaglia L, Perino A, Hamou J. Hysteroscopy in perimenopausal and postmenopausal women with abnormal uterine bleeding. J Reprod Med 1987; 32:577–582.
8. Kaunitz AM. Abnormal uterine bleeding in the perimenopausal patient. Contemp OB/GYN 2002; April:69–88.
9. Kilbourn CL, Richards CS. Abnormal uterine bleeding—diagnostic considerations, management options. Postgrad Med 2001; 109:1–11.
10. Munro MG. Abnormal uterine bleeding in the reproductive years. Part I—pathogenesis and clinical investigation. J Am Assoc Gynecol Laparosc 1999; 6:391–418.
11. Kurman RJ, Kaminski PF, Norris HJ. The behavior of endometrial hyperplasia—A long-term study of untreated hyperplasia in 170 patients. Cancer 1988; 56:403–412.
12. Farquhar CM, Lethaby A, Sowter M et al. An evaluation of risk factors for endometrial hyperplasia in premenopausal women with abnormal menstrual bleeding. Am J Obstet Gynecol 1999; 181:525–529.

13. Nichols WC, Ginsburg D. von Willebrand disease. Medicine 1997; 76:1–20.
14. Dilley A, Drews C, Miller C. von Willebrand disease and other inherited bleeding disorders in women diagnosed with menorrhagia. Obstet Gynecol 2001; 97:630–636.
15. March CM. Bleeding problems and treatment. Clin Obstet Gynecol 1998; 41:928–939.
16. Rodin DA, Bano G, Bland JM et al. Polycystic ovaries and associated metabolic abnormalities in Indian subcontinent Asian women. Clin Endocrinol (Oxf) 1998; 49:91–99.
17. Lusker JM. Screening and diagnosis of coagulation disorders. Am J Obstet Gynecol 1996; 175:778–783.
18. Grimes DA. Diagnostic dilation and curettage: A reappraisal. Am J Obstet Gynecol 1982; 142:1–6.
19. Smith JJ, Schulman H. Current dilation and curettage practice: A need for revision. Am J Obstet Gynecol 1985; 65:516–518.
20. Stovall TG, Solomon SK, Ling FW. Endometrial sampling prior to hysterectomy. Obstet Gynecol 1989; 73:405–409.
21. MacKenzie IZ, Bibby JG. Critical assessment of dilatation and curettage in 1029 women. Lancet 1978; 2:566–568.
22. Stovall TG, Ling FW, Morgan PL. A prospective, randomized comparison of the pipelle endometrial sampling device with the Novak curette. Am J Obstet Gynecol 1991; 165:1287–1290.
23. Stovall TG, Photopulos GJ, Poston WM et al. Pipelle endometrial sampling in patients with known endometrial carcinoma. Obstet Gynecol 1991; 77:954–956.
24. Smith-Brindham R, Kerlikowske K, Felstein VA. Endovaginal ultrasound to exclude endometrial cancer and other endometrial abnormalities. JAMA 1998; 280:1510–1517.
25. Tabor A, Watt HC, Wald NJ. Endometrial thickness as a test for endometrial cancer in women with postmenopausal bleeding. Obstet Gynecol 2002; 99:663–670.
26. Goldstein SR, Zeltser I, Horan CK et al. Ultrasonography-based triage for perimenopausal patients with abnormal uterine bleeding. Am J Obstet Gynecol 1997; 177:102–108.
27. Dijkhuizen FP, DeVries LD, Mol BW et al. Comparison of transvaginal ultrasonography and saline infusion sonography for the detection of intracavitary abnormalities in premenopausal women. Ultrasound Obstet Gynecol 2000; 15:372–376.
28. Dueholm M, Forman A, Jensen ML et al. Transvaginal sonography combined with saline contrast sonohysterography in evaluating the uterine cavity in premenopausal patients with abnormal uterine bleeding. Ultrasound Obstet Gynecol 2001; 18:54–61.
29. Deuholm M, Jensen ML, Laursen H et al. Can the endometrial thickness as measured by transvaginal sonography be used to exclude polyps or hyperplasia in premenopausal patients with abnormal uterine bleeding. Acta Obstet Gynecol Scand 2001; 80:645–651.
30. Widrich T, Bradley LD, Mitchinson AR et al. Comparison of saline infusion sonography with office hysteroscopy for evaluation of the endometrium. Am J Obstet Gynecol 1996; 174:1327–1334.
31. Bernard JP, Rizk E, Comattes S et al. Saline contrast sonohysterography in the preoperative assessment of benign intrauterine disorders. Ultrasound Obstet Gynecol 2001; 17:145–149.
32. Di Naro E, Bratta FG, Romano F. The diagnosis of benign uterine pathology using transvaginal endohysterosonography. Clin Exp Obstet Gynecol 1996; 23:103–107.
33. Parsons AK, Lense JJ. Sonohysterography for endometrial abnormalities: Preliminary results. J Clin Ultrasound 1993; 21:87–95.
34. Clevenger-Hoeft M, Syrop CH, Stovall DW et al. Sonohysterography in premenopausal women with and without abnormal bleeding. Obstet Gynecol 1999; 94:516–520.
35. Hidlebaugh DH. Comparison of clinical outcomes and cost of office versus hospital hysteroscopy. J Am Assoc Gynecol Laparosc 1996; 4:39–45.
36. Jansen FW, Vredevoogd CB, Van Ulzen K. Complications of hysteroscopy: A prospective multicenter study. Obstet Gynecol 2000; 96:266–270.
37. Zerbe MJ, Zhang J, Bristow RE. Retrograde seeding of malignant cells during hysteroscopy in presumed early endometrial cancer. Gynecol Oncol 2000; 79:55–58.
38. Obermair A, Geramou M, Gucer F. Impact of hysteroscopy on disease-free survival in clinically stage I endometrial cancer patients. Int J Gynecol Cancer 2000; 10:275–279.

39. Vercellini P, Cortesi I, DeGiorgi O. Transvaginal ultrasonography versus uterine needle biopsy in the diagnosis of diffuse adenomyosis. Human Reprod 1998; 13:2884–2887.

40. Lethaby A, Augood C, Duckitt K. Nonsteroidal anti-inflammatory drugs for heavy menstrual bleeding (Cochrane Review). In Cochrane Library 2002; Issue 1. Oxford: Update Software.

41. Munro MG. Abnormal uterine bleeding in the reproductive years. Part II—Medical Management. J Am Assoc Gynecol Laparosc 2000; (1):17–34.

42. Lethaby A, Farquhar C, Cooke I. Antifibrinolytics for heavy menstrual bleeding (Cochrane Review). In Cochrane Library 2002; Issue 2. Oxford: Update Software.

43. Lindoff C, Rybo G, Astedt B. Treatment with tranexamic acid during pregnancy and risk of thrombo-embolic complications. Throm Haemost 1993; 70(2):238–240.

44. Kaunitz AM. Oral contraceptive use in perimenopause. Am J Obstet Gynecol 2001; 185 (2 Suppl):532–537.

45. Fraser IS, McGarron G: Randomized trial of 2 hormonal and 2 prostaglandin-inhibiting agents in women with a complaint of menorrhagia. Aust N ZJ Obstet Gynaecol 1991; 31 (1):66–70.

46. Davis A, Godwin A, Lippman J et al. Triphasic norgestimate-ethinyl estradiol for treating dysfunctional uterine bleeding. Obstet Gynecol 2000; 96:913–920.

47. Casper RF, Dodin S, Reid RL et al. The effect of 20 mg ethinyl estradiol/1 mg norethindrone acetate (Minestrin), a low-dose oral contraceptive on vaginal bleeding patterns, hot flashes, and quality of life in symptomatic perimenopausal women. Menopause 1997; 4:139–147.

48. Carr BR, Ory H. Estrogen and progestin components of oral contraceptives: Relationship to vascular disease. Contraception 1997; 55:267–272.

49. Nightingale AL, Lawrenson RA, Simpson EL et al. The effects of age, body mass index, smoking and general health on the risk of venous thrombo-embolism in users of combined oral contraceptives. Eur J Contracept Reprod Health Care 2000; 5:265–274.

50. Baerug U, Winge T, Nordland G. Do combinations of 1 mg estradiol and low doses of NETA effectively control menopausal symptoms? Climacteric 1998; 1:219–228.

51. Stadberg E, Mattson LA, Uvebrant M. 17 beta-estradiol and norethisterone acetate in low doses as continuous combined hormone replacement therapy. Maturitas 1996; 23:31–39.

52. Williams SR, Frenchek B, Speroff L. A study of combined continuous ethinyl estradiol and norethindrone acetate for postmenopausal hormone replacement. Am J Obstet Gynecol 1990; 162:438–446.

53. Archer DF, Dorin MH, Heine W et al. Uterine bleeding in postmenopausal women on continuous therapy with estradiol and norethindrone acetate. Endometrium study group. Obstet Gynecol 1999; 94:323–329.

54. Speroff L. Management of the perimenopausal transition. Contemporary OB/GYN 2000; 45:14–37.

55. Lethaby AE, Cooke I, Rees M. Progesterone/progestogen releasing intrauterine system versus either placebo or any other medication for heavy menstrual bleeding. (Cochrane Review). In Cochrane Library 2002; Issue 1. Oxford: Update Software.

56. Hurskainen R, Teperi J, Rissenen P et al. Quality of life and cost-effectiveness of levonorgestrel-releasing intrauterine system versus hysterectomy for treatment of menorrhagia: A randomized trial. Lancet 2001; 357:273–277.

57. Goldrath MH. Use of Danazol in Hysteroscopic surgery for menorrhagia. J Reprod Med 1990; 35:91–96.

58. Schlaff WD, Zerhouni EA, Huth JA et al. A placebo-controlled trial of a depot gonadotropin-releasing hormone analogue (leuprolide) in the treatment of uterine leiomyomata. Obstet Gynecol 1989; 74:856–862.

59. Friedman AJ, Hoffman DI, Comite F et al. Treatment of leiomyomata with leuprolide acetate depot: A double-blind placebo-controlled, multicenter study. Leuprolide Study Group. Obstet Gynecol 1991; 77:720–725.

60. DeVore GR, Owens O, Kase N. Use of intravenous Premarin in the treatment of dysfunctional uterine bleeding—a double-blind randomized control study. Obstet Gynecol 1982; 59:285–291.

61. Lepina LA, Hillis SD, Marchbarks PA et al. Hysterectomy surveillance—United States, 1980–1993. Mor Mortal Wkly Rep CDC Surveill Summ 1997; 46:1–15.

62. Kozak LJ, Lawrence L. National hospital discharge: Annual summary 1997. Vital Health Stat 1999; i–iv; 1–46.
63. Vercellini P, Zaina B, Yaylayan L et al. Hysteroscopic myomectomy: Long-term effects on menstrual pattern and fertility. Obstet Gynecol 1999; 94:341–347.
64. Hallez JP. Single-stage total hysteroscopic myomectomies: Indications, techniques and results. Fertil Steril 1995; 63:703–708.
65. Goldrath MH, Fuller TA, Segal S. Laser photovaporization of endometrium for the treatment of menorrhagia. Am J Obstet Gynecol 1981; 140:14–19.
66. Weber AM. Endometrial ablation. Obstet Gynecol 2002; 99(6):969–970.
67. Boujida VH, Philipsen T, Pelle J et al. Five-year follow-up of endometrial ablation: Endometrial coagulation versus endometrial resection. Obstet Gynecol 2002; 99:988–992.
68. Munro MG. Abnormal uterine bleeding: Surgical management—Part III. J Am Assoc Gynecol Laparosc 2001; 7(4):18–47.
69. Lethaby A, Sheppard S, Cooke I et al. Endometrial resection and ablation versus hysterectomy for heavy menstrual bleeding (Cochrane Review). In Cochrane Library 2002; Issue 1 Oxford: Update Software.
70. Baggish MS, Sze EH. Endometrial ablation: A series of 568 patients treated over an 11-year period. Am J Obstet Gynecol 1996; 174:908–913.
71. Vercellini P, Oldani S, Yaylayan L et al. Randomized comparison of vaporizing electrode and cutting loop for endometrial ablation. Obstet Gynecol 1999; 94:521–527.
72. Meyer WR, Walsh BW, Grainger DA et al. Thermal balloon and rollerball ablation to treat menorrhagia: A multicenter comparison. Obstet Gynecol 1998; 92:98–103.
73. Grainger DA, Tjaden BL, Rowland C et al. Thermal balloon and rollerball ablation to treat menorrhagia: Two-year results of a multicenter, prospective, randomized clinical trial. J Am Assoc Gynecol Laparosc 2000; 7:175–179.
74. Bongers MY, Mol BW, Brolmann HA. Prognostic factors for success of thermal balloon ablation in the treatment of menorrhagia. Obstet Gynecol 2002; 99:1060–1066.
75. das Dores GB, Richart RM, Nicolau SM et al. Evaluation of hydro thermoblator for endometrial destruction in patients with menorrhagia. J Am Assoc Gynecol Laparosc 1999; 6:275–278.
76. Corson SL. A multicenter evaluation of endometrial ablation by Hydrotherm Ablator and rollerball for treatment of menorrhagia. J Am Assoc Gynecol Laparosc 2001; 8:359–367.
77. Bain C, Cooper KG, Parkin DE. Microwave endometrial ablation versus endometrial resection: A randomized controlled trial. Obstet Gynecol 2002; 99:983–987.
78. Sowter MC, Singla AA, Lethaby A. Pre-operative endometrial thinning agents before hysteroscopic surgery for heavy menstrual bleeding (Cochrane Review). In Cochrane Library 2002; Issue 1. Oxford: Update Software.
79. Alexander DA, Naji AA, Pinion SB et al. Randomised trial comparing hysterectomy with endometrial ablation for dysfunctional uterine bleeding: Psychiatric and psychosocial aspects. BMJ 1996; 312:280–284.
80. Broder MS, Kanouse DE, Mittman BS et al. The appropriateness of recommendations for hysterectomy. Obstet Gynecol 2000; 95:199–205.
81. Lethaby A, Vollenhouen B, Sowter M. Pre-operative GnRH analogue therapy before hysterectomy or myomectomy for uterine fibroids. (Cochrane Review). In: Cochrane Library 2000, Issue 3. Oxford: Update Software.
82. Stovall TG, Ling FW, Henry LC et al. A randomized trial evaluating leuprolide acetate before hysterectomy as treatment for leiomyomas. Am J Obstet Gynecol 1991; 164:1420–1425.
83. Worthington-Kirsch RL, Popky GL, Hutchins FLJ. Uterine artery embolization for the management of leiomyomas: Quality-of-life assessment and clinical response. Radiology 1998; 208:625–629.
84. Young AE, Malinak LR, Harper A et al. Uterine artery embolization for the treatment of symptomatic leiomyomata. Obstet Gynecol 2000; 95(4 suppl 1):526.
85. Johnston BA. One-third of nation's adults use herbal remedies. Herbal Gram 1997; 40:49.
86. Knight DC, Eden JA. Phytoestrogens—A short review. Maturitas 1995; 22:167–175.

87. Rose DP, Boyer AP, Wynder EL. International comparison of mortality rates for cancer of the breast, ovary, prostate, and colon, per capita fa consumption. Cancer 1986; 58:2363–2371.

88. Parkin DM. Cancers of the breast, endometrium, and ovary. Geographical correlations. Eur J Cancer Clin Oncol 1989; 25:1917–1925.

89. Israel D, Youngkin EQ. Herbal therapies for perimenopausal and menopausal complaints. Pharmacotherapy 1997; 17 (5):970–984.

90. Zhang Y, Wang X. 50 cases of dysfunctional uterine bleeding treated by puncturing the effective points—A new system of acupuncture. J of Trad Chin Med 1994; 14(4):287–291.

91. Fessenden JM, Wittenborn W, Clarke L et al. A case report of herbal medicine and bleeding postoperatively from a laparoscopic cholecystectomy. Am Surg 2001; 67(1):3–35.

92. Gianni LM, Dreitlein WB. Some popular OTC herbals can interact with anticoagulant therapy. US Pharmacist 1998; 23(80):83–84.

3

Fertility Issues of the Perimenopause

R. Stan Williams
Department of Obstetrics and Gynecology,
University of Florida College of Medicine, Gainesville, Florida, U.S.A.

I. AGE AND FERTILITY

Infertility is a common condition affecting 10% to 15% of couples. As the baby boom generation has aged, the demand for infertility services has grown substantially. Many women of the baby boom generation have delayed childbearing in order to pursue professional careers and as a consequence are starting families in their fourth decade of life. Between 1990 and 2000, one out of every five women was having her first child after age 35, a 50% increase compared to previous years (1). The prevalence of infertility almost doubles from ages 30 to 34 to ages 35 to 39, from 15% up to 25% to 30% respectively. Several etiologic factors increase the risk of infertility with advancing female age including increased lifetime risk of developing pelvic inflammatory disease, endometriosis, pelvic surgery, environmental factors, and lifestyle factors such as smoking and alcohol intake. Even controlling for these factors, however, increasing female age has a dramatic inverse relationship to fertility (2) (Fig. 1).

Studies that have compared natural fertility rates in populations that do not practice contraception such as the Hutterites, show a gradual decline of female fertility between ages 30 to 35 with a much steeper decline after age 35 and particularly after age 40 (3).

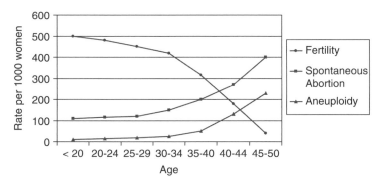

Figure 1 With increasing maternal age, there is a dramatic decrease in fertility rates and increase in spontaneous abortion rates and aneuploidy rates.

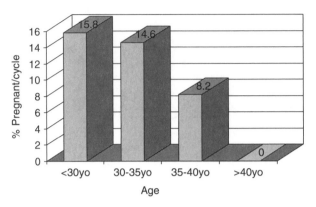

Figure 2 Cycle pregnancy rates at the University of Florida in women using donor sperm, by maternal age.

These declines of fertility are mirrored in other demographic studies of populations in the nineteenth and twentieth centuries (4).

Several studies of donor insemination have also dramatically demonstrated the effect of advancing female age on achieving a successful pregnancy (1,5,6). These donor insemination studies eliminate the variable of decreasing sexual activity with advancing age of couples and male factor infertility. At the University of Florida, cycle pregnancy rates with the use of donor insemination were 16% in women less than 30 years of age, 15% between ages 30 and 35, 8% between ages 36 and 40, and with a limited number of cycles, 0% in women over age 40 (6) (Fig. 2).

The most dramatic illustration of female age on pregnancy success is seen in couples undergoing in vitro fertilization (IVF). In 1999, U.S. national statistics for all IVF centers show that birth rates among women in their twenties and early thirties were relatively stable at approximately 32%, but declined steadily in women aged up to 35. At age 40, birth rates were approximately 15% and by age 44, less than 5% (7).

In addition to declining fertility rates, age is also associated with increasing spontaneous abortion rates, as well as an increasing incidence of chromosomal aneuploidy (8). While women at age 20 have an incidence of one in 2000 of having a live born infant with a chromosomal aneuploidy, by age 35 this has risen to one in 200, and by age 40 one in 80. Even more profound than the chromosomal aneuploidy rate in live births is the aneuploidy rate recognized in embryos. In vitro fertilization studies have shown that aneuploidy rates exceed 50% in embryos that were fertilized in vitro and is increased in patients with advancing reproductive age (9, 10).

Increasing aneuploidy rates are thought to be responsible for the increasing spontaneous abortion rate seen with advancing maternal age. Even after cardiac activity has been documented by ultrasound, the spontaneous abortion rate varies dramatically for differing maternal ages (9). A spontaneous abortion rate of 2% was observed for maternal ages less than 35 after documentation of cardiac activity by ultrasound, but this rate increased to 16% for patients older than 36 and to 20% for women older than 40. (Fig. 3).

Until recently, there has been a debate about whether ovarian or uterine factors are the principal cause for the age-related decline in fertility. A number of age-related uterine and endometrial changes have been seen in other animal species, but has not been substantiated in humans. With the advent of in vitro fertilization and donor egg programs, we have an excellent model for examining the contribution to fertility success of both the uterus and oocyte. By comparing success rates of in vitro fertilization with eggs donated from young women placed into the uterus of older women, the age effects of each can be separated. In the

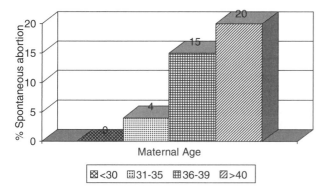

Figure 3 The incidence of spontaneous abortion after cardiac activity is identified by ultrasound varies by maternal age. *Source:* From Ref. 9.

United States in 1999, live birth rates per embryo transfer in women using donor eggs was stable from age 30 through age 46 at approximately 40%. In contrast, the live birth rate per transfer when using their own eggs experienced a significant decline after age 35 (7) (Fig. 4). This observation clearly demonstrates that it is the age of the woman donating the egg and not the age of the uterus, which is most critical in reproductive outcome. Similarly, spontaneous abortion rates and aneuploidy are primarily dependent on the age of the egg donor (2).

Although advancing age is clearly associated with a decline of reproductive success, the relative contribution of nuclear versus cytoplasmic changes within the aging oocyte is unknown. It is known that there is a higher frequency of abnormal meiotic spindle formation in oocytes from older women. The meiotic spindle is composed of microtubules, which assembles outside the cell nucleus. It is thought that damage in these microtubules and associated proteins would lead to abnormal segregation of chromosomes during meiosis. An attempt to repair this defect by injecting donor cytoplasm into an aged recipient oocyte has resulted in successful pregnancy (11). Whether the cytoplasmic transfer was responsible for the successful pregnancy is unknown. Currently, work in this area has been halted because cytoplasmic transfer involves the transfer of mitochondrial DNA and the FDA has prohibited any procedure which would result in the transfer of DNA to offspring since this could be viewed as a type of cloning. Alternatively, it is reasonable to suspect

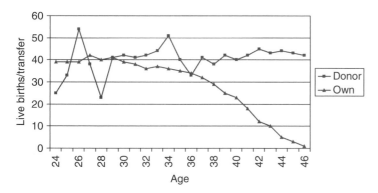

Figure 4 National IVF success rates in 1999 illustrating the dramatic decline of success with advancing maternal age when using their own age, but in age independent success when using eggs from young donors. *Source:* From Ref. 7.

that with advancing age the oocyte can acquire damage to its chromosomes and DNA which may not be repaired properly and would result in chromosomally abnormal oocytes and embryos.

Reproductive aging is also associated with declining number of primordial follicles and accelerated follicular development. The rate of decline of primordial follicles is thought to be stable until approximately age 38 when an acceleration in primordial follicle depletion begins (12). This process may be accelerated by elevated follicle-stimulating harmone (FSH) levels, which are a marker for decreased ovarian reserve and are increased as women age. These higher FSH levels are also thought to accelerate dominant follicle development and lead to shorter menstrual cycles, which are associated with declining fertility (13). Women aged 40 to 45 have a higher early follicular phase FSH than women aged 20 to 25 (12). The basis for this FSH rise is a decrease in inhibin B production in the early follicular phase and perhaps a decrease in inhibin A in the luteal phase, as well as increasing activin A levels. All these changes are associated with declining oocyte complex function (14–18) (Fig. 5).

II. OVARIAN RESERVE TESTING

The relatively wide age of normal menopause, 42 to 58 years (mean +/− two standard deviations), indicates that aging of the ovary and primordial follicles occurs at dramatically different rates in individual women. Thus, some women will have declining fertility prior to age 35 while others will maintain normal fertility into their forties. Since women lose their fertility at different rates, there has been an attempt to devise biochemical and morphological markers for normal fertility status, usually referred to as ovarian reserve.

An abnormal rise in early follicular phase FSH levels measured on cycle day 2, 3, or 4, has been associated with declining ovarian response to gonadotropin stimulation and low pregnancy rates. Toner et al. studied 1478 consecutive IVF cycles and the ability of a day 3 FSH level and age to predict IVF success rates (19). They concluded that day 3 FSH was

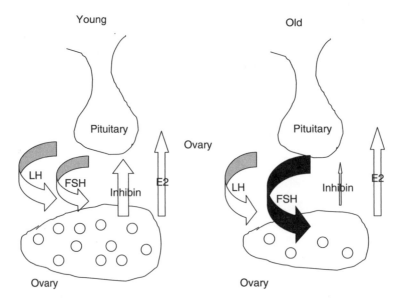

Figure 5 As maternal age increases the reduction in follicle number, as well as reduction in aging of the remaining follicles produces a decline of inhibin. The lack of inhibin feedback at the pituitary results in an increase of FSH while estradiol levels remain unchanged.

a better single predictor than age for pregnancy success. When FSH levels were greater than 25 IU/ml (as measured by Leeco RIA), they had no ongoing pregnancies at any age. A number of other investigators have confirmed that elevated day 3 FSH values are correlated with extremely low pregnancy rates in IVF patients, after controlling for the age of the patient (1,20,21). Advancing age, however, remains an important independent determinate of IVF success with increased age being associated with poor stimulation, more cancellation cycles, less transfers, less pregnancies and more miscarriages. Both the age of the female, as well as her basal FSH status should be taken into account when trying to predict reproductive success.

Investigators have also examined early follicular estradiol levels in association with early follicular FSH and have determined that elevated estradiol levels are associated with a poor prognosis of pregnancy (2,21,22). Premature estradiol elevation suggests early recruitment of follicles secondary to elevated gonadotropins in the late luteal phase of the preceding cycle with accelerated follicular maturation and follicular dominance. Estradiol levels above 50 to 75 pg/ml are associated with a poor chance of pregnancy even with a normal day 3 FSH. The elevated estradiol at this time artificially suppresses FSH to a normal level so in the face of an elevated estradiol, the basal FSH value cannot be interpreted properly.

Basal levels of FSH may vary from cycle to cycle. In patients with normal ovarian reserve, the variation averages 2 to 3 mIU/ml whereas in patients with poor ovarian reserve, the variability is more marked with a mean deviation of 7 to 8 mIU/ml (23). Despite initiation of treatment in cycles with normal basal FSH values, patients identified as having large intercycle variations of their basal FSH value continue to respond poorly to gonadotropin stimulation and have poor reproductive outcomes. A poor prognosis can be anticipated in patients who have ever demonstrated elevated basal FSH values and had normal levels in subsequent cycles. Thus continued monitoring of their FSH values is unwarranted.

Basal FSH values have been compared in women with 1 versus 2 ovaries. Women who have had a prior oophorectomy are more likely to have elevated basal FSH values. However, in such women with normal basal FSH values, the chance of pregnancy was no different from those women with two ovaries (22,24).

Elevated day 3 FSH has not only been associated with poor response to stimulation and reduced likelihood of pregnancy, but has also been associated with a significantly higher chance of abnormal fetal karyotype (25). Women with an elevated day 3 FSH or estradiol were found to be more likely to have a karyotypically abnormal spontaneous abortion than women with normal basal values. The most common abnormality noted was autosomal trisomy (79.5%).

III. CLOMIPHENE CITRATE CHALLENGE TEST

The clomiphene citrate challenge test (CCCT) is a provocative test which includes a basal day 3 FSH level. If the day 3 FSH is normal it is followed by clomiphene citrate 100 mg daily from cycle days 5 to 9. A second FSH value is obtained on day 10. The test is considered abnormal if either the day 3 or day 10 FSH value is elevated above the value for normal ovarian reserve (2,21,22). Navot et al., in their initial report, studied 51 women aged 35 years or more with unexplained infertility who all had normal day 3 FSH values. Eighteen of these women exhibited abnormal day 10 FSH values and only one of these conceived (26). Other reports have confirmed the predictive value of an abnormal CCCT with an overall cumulative pregnancy rate of only 1.3% (2,27). The CCCT is able to identify a significantly larger population of patients with abnormal ovarian reserve when compared with basal FSH screening alone. In women over age 35, the CCCT will identify

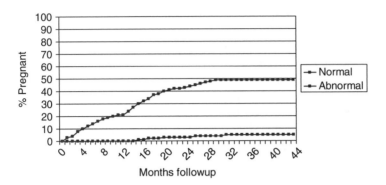

Figure 6 Pregnancy rates regardless of age are extremely low in women who have had an abnormal Clomid challenge test in a general infertility population. *Source:* From Ref. 27.

approximately 30% of women with compromised fertility compared with only 6% detection rate for basal FSH screening alone (2). Using the CCCT instead of only measuring day 3 FSH will markedly increase the sensitivity of identifying women with poor ovarian reserve.

The CCCT has also been studied in a general infertility population. Scott et al. followed 588 women over 45 months after a thorough infertility evaluation and appropriate treatment. Women with an abnormal CCCT had a poor pregnancy rate independent of age. However, age remained an important prognostic factor in determining pregnancy success in women with a normal CCCT (28,29) (Fig. 6). The continued decline of fertility seen with advancing age despite a normal clomiphene citrate challenge test emphasizes that there are other factors impacting pregnancy success that are not measured by the CCCT. In women with an abnormal CCCT, their chance of pregnancy over almost four years of treatment and follow-up was approximately 5%.

The CCCT has been proposed as the most sensitive measure of diminished ovarian reserve and poor prognosis for pregnancy (22). Ovarian reserve screening with the CCCT should be considered in women over age 35, women with unexplained infertility, and women with a poor stimulation using gonadotropins. Despite a normal CCCT, women will experience significant declines of their fertility in their late thirties and early forties. Thus, age should be used as an independent but related prognostic factor. Women who smoke are also at increased risk for decreased ovarian reserve when compared with age matched controls as detected by the CCCT (30).

IV. VARIABILITY IN DIFFERENT FSH ASSAYS

FSH and LH are glycoprotein hormones composed of a common alpha chain and unique beta chains. The protein backbone is produced with a variable degree of glycosylation. The glycosylation of these proteins can vary depending on the hormonal milieu and will thus differ throughout the menstrual cycle. Glycosylation impacts both the bioactivity of these hormones and their half-lives, but also significantly influences their measurement by hormone assays.

Different antibodies to measure FSH have been developed by different commercial assay systems. These polyclonal antibodies bind differently to separate regions on the glycoprotein hormones and significant differences in these polyclonal antibodies exist between assay systems. Consequently, because of the differing isoforms of FSH produced throughout the menstrual cycle and the different antibody systems developed by commercial assays, comparison of results between assay systems is extremely difficult (22).

The original descriptions of elevated basal FSH values used a Leeco RIA system with a threshold for normal ovarian reserve at 25 mIU/ml. More recent ELISA assays have been reported to have abnormal ovarian reserve with thresholds of FSH as low as 10 mIU/ml (21,22). Practically, this means that one should validate the results of each laboratory for abnormal ovarian reserve FSH thresholds instead of using published FSH thresholds. One could anticipate that FSH assays using RIA technology would be more likely to have thresholds between 20 and 25 mIU/ml, whereas assays using more recently developed ELISA tests would have thresholds between 10 and 15 mIU/ml. It should be noted that ovarian reserve values are significantly lower than thresholds that laboratories report as menopausal (usually > 40).

V. GnRH AGONIST STIMULATION TEST (GAST)

Another approach to detecting the status of ovarian reserve has utilized changes in estradiol after administration of leuprolide acetate (31), a GnRH agonist. Leuprolide acetate 1 mg subcutaneously was given on cycle day 2 and estradiol measured before the agonist was administered and 24 hours after the agonist. In the setting of IVF, the magnitude of increase of estradiol correlated strongly with success. This test has not been validated outside of IVF and its applicability to the general infertility population would be both more expensive and somewhat more invasive. It is not known how the predictability of the gonadotropin releasing hormone agonist stimulation test, or GAST, compares with the CCCT.

VI. INHIBIN

Inhibin is a heterodimeric glycoprotein consisting of alpha and one of two beta subunits (β a and β b), which when combined with the alpha subunit form inhibin A and inhibin B respectively. Inhibin is produced by the granulosa cells, and as the name implies, is known to inhibit the pituitary release of FSH. Since it has been observed that estradiol levels are usually within the normal range in the early follicular phase despite elevated basal FSH values, it was hypothesized that the rise in FSH seen with reproductive aging was secondary to diminishing production of inhibin by the compromised oocyte granulosa complex (32,33,12). Follicular phase inhibin B levels and luteal phase inhibin A levels are inversely correlated with advancing age (33). Using a dimeric inhibin assay, Seifer demonstrated that if inhibin B measured on cycle day 3 was less than 45 pg/ml controlling for age, day 3 FSH and day 3 E2, subjects had a poor response to ovulation induction and a poor prognosis to clinical pregnancy with IVF (32).

Clinical use of inhibin B as a predictor of ovarian reserve will depend on widespread availability of accurate commercial assays and further research into the applicability of inhibin assays in the general population.

VII. ULTRASOUND MEASUREMENTS OF THE OVARIAN FOLLICLE POOL

Observations show that follicle numbers decline in a biexponential fashion with age, with an increased rate of declining follicles after age 38. Attempts have been made to use ultrasound measurements of the ovary and early antral follicles as predictors of reproductive success (34). Since measurements of the ovary by transvaginal ultrasound are consistent between observers (35), measurements of both ovarian volume and antral follicle count have been used as non-invasive, simple predictors of ovarian reserve.

In 1995 Syrop et al. reported a retrospective evaluation of 188 women undergoing IVF (36). Total ovarian volume (right plus left ovarian volumes), as well as the volume of the smallest ovary were calculated in pretreatment IVF transvaginal ultrasounds. Ovarian volume was measured using a formula for an ellipse, 0.526 (length × height × width). The pregnancy rate decreased from 46% to 28% when the volume of the smallest ovary decreased from greater than 9 cm^3 to less than 3 cm^3. Using total ovarian volume, clinical pregnancy rates decreased from 50% to 31% when total ovarian volume was greater than 22 cm^3 versus less than 8.6 cm^3 (36). Similarly, Lass et al. demonstrated in 140 women undergoing IVF that an ovarian volume of less than 3 cm^3 was associated with a very high cycle cancellation rate, 53%, compared to a group with normal ovarian volume, 9%. These authors reported an association with increasing age and smaller ovarian volumes but all patients in this study had normal day 3 FSH values. Patients who had embryo transfers in the small ovarian volume group had no difference in their fertilization or pregnancy rates compared to the normal ovarian volume group (37). Both of these earlier studies have been confirmed by other groups (38,39). Thus, measurement of ovarian volume seems to be a predictor of decreased ovarian reserve primarily seen as a poor response to gonadotropin stimulation and higher treatment cancellation rates.

A correlation of follicle density and early follicular FSH values has been demonstrated by ovarian biopsy (40). Ultrasound has also been used to assess the declining ovarian follicle pool. The decreasing number of follicles seen with advancing age can also be measured by transvaginal ultrasound examining early antral follicles measuring 2 to 5 mm (Fig. 7). In 31 healthy women, the number of antral follicles decreased by about 60% between ages 22 and 42 (41). Subsequently, Tomas et al. reported on 166 women undergoing IVF. They found that in women with less than five early antral follicles prior to stimulation, significantly fewer numbers of oocytes were recovered. The antral follicle count was a better predictor of stimulation outcome than was ovarian volume when controlled for age (42). Other investigators have also described the correlation between low antral

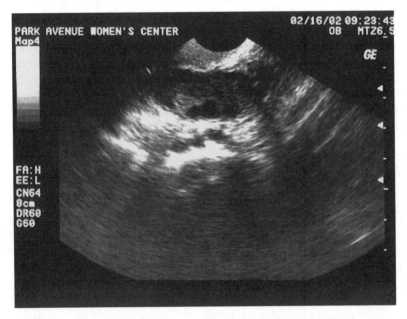

Figure 7 A transvaginal ultrasound in the early follicular phase demonstrating early antral follicles measuring 2–5 mm.

follicle numbers (<3–5) and poor response to stimulation, higher rates of cycle cancellation, and poor pregnancy outcome (43,44,45).

Although ultrasound measurements have been primarily used to predict IVF outcomes, it would seem logical that these measurements may also predict ovarian reserve status in the general population. Until these studies are performed, however, transvaginal ultrasound measurement of ovarian volume and early antral follicle formation will primarily be a tool for IVF programs so that they may prospectively be able to determine the best stimulation protocols and to inform the patient of their expected success.

VIII. SUMMARY FOR OVARIAN RESERVE SCREENING

At the current time the best characterized and most sensitive test for ovarian reserve is the clomiphene citrate challenge test. This test has been studied both in the general infertility population, as well as in women undergoing IVF. It has an increased sensitivity over basal day 3 FSH levels and has a strongly predictive value when abnormal. Independently, age should also strongly be considered as a measure of ovarian reserve if the clomiphene citrate challenge test is normal. These tests, however, do not have absolute specificity or sensitivity and although patients should be counseled about their chances of conception, they should not be informed that pregnancy is not possible. They may, however, want to strongly consider alternatives such as oocyte donation to maximize their chance of conception.

REFERENCES

1. American Society for Reproductive Medicine, Guideline for Practice, Age Related Infertility.
2. Klein J, Sauer MV. Assessing fertility in women of advanced reproductive age. AJOG Reviews, 2001; 185(3):758–770.
3. Tietze C. Reproductive span and rate of reproduction among hutterite women. Fertility and Sterility, 1957; 8(1):89–97.
4. Menken J, Trussell J, Larsen U. Age and infertility. Science, 1986; 233(4771):1389–1394.
5. Virro MR, Shewchuk AB. Pregnancy outcome in 242 conceptions after artificial insemination with donor sperm and effects of maternal age on the prognosis for successful pregnancy. Am J Obstet Gynecol, 1984; 148(5):518–524.
6. Williams RS, Alderman J. Predictors of success with the use of donor sperm. Am J Obstet Gynecol, 2001; 185(2):332–337.
7. 1999 Assisted Reproductive Technology Success Rates. National Summary and Fertility Clinic Reports.
8. Hassold T, Jacobs P, Kline J et al. Effect of maternal age on autosomal trisomies. Ann Hum Genet, 1980; 44(Pt1):29–36.
9. Smith KE, Buyalos RP. The profound impact of patient age on pregnancy outcome after early detection of fetal cardiac activity. Fertility and Sterility, 1996; 65(4):35–40.
10. Munne S, Grifo J, Alikani M et al. Embryo morphology, developmental rates, and maternal age are correlated with chromosome abnormalities. Fertility and Sterility, 1995; 64(2):382–391.
11. Cohen J, Scott R, Schimmel T et al. Birth of an infant after transfer of a nucleate donor oocyte cytoplasm into recipient eggs. Lancet 1997; 350(9072):186–187.
12. Klein NA, Soules MR. Menopausal Medicine. Summer: ASRM Newsletter 1999:9–12.
13. Klein NA, Battaglia DE, Fujimoto VY et al. Reproductive aging: Accelerated ovarian follicular development associated with a monotropic follicle-stimulating hormone rise in normal older women. Journal of Clinical Endocrinology and Metabolism, 1996; 81(3):1038–1045.
14. Lee SJ, Lenton EA, Sexton L et al. The effect of age on the cyclical patterns of plasma LH, FSH, oestradiol and progesterone in women with regular menstrual cycles. IRL Press Limited, 1988; 3(7):851–855.

15. Soules MR, Battaglia DE, Klein NA. Inhibin and reproductive aging in women. The European Menopause Journal, 1998; 30(2):193–204.

16. Santoro N, Rosenberg-Brown J et al. Characterization of reproductive hormonal dynamics in the perimenopause. Journal of Clinical Endocrinology and Metabolism, 1996; 81(4):1495–1501.

17. Klein NA, Illingworth PJ, Groome NP et al. Decreased inhibin B secretion is associated with the monotropic FSH rise in older, ovulatory women: A study of serum and follicular fluid levels of dimeric inhibin A and B in spontaneous menstrual cycles. Journal of clinical endocrinology and metabolism, 1996; 81(7):2742–2745.

18. Reame NE, Wyman TL, Phillips DJ et al. Net increase in stimulatory input resulting from a decrease in inhibin B and an increase in activin A may contribute in part to the rise in follicular phase follicle-stimulating hormone of aging cycling women. Journal of Clinical Endocrinology and Metabolism, 1998; 83(9):3302–3307.

19. Toner JP, Philput CB, Jones GS et al. Basal follicle-stimulating hormone level is a better predictor of in vitro fertilization performance than age. Fertility and Sterility, 1991; 56(3):784–791.

20. Pearlstone AC, Pang SC, Fournet N et al. Ovulation induction in women age 40 and older: The importance of basal follicle-stimulating hormone level and chronological age. Fertility and Sterility, 1992; 58(4):674–679.

21. Toner JP, Scott RT. Chronologic versus ovarian age impact on pregnancy among infertile couples. seminars in reproductive endocrinology, 1995:1–15.

22. Scott RT, Hofmann GE. Prognostic assessment of ovarian reserve. Fertility and Sterility, 1995; 63(1):1–11.

23. Scott RT, Hofmann GE, Oehninger, S et al. Intercycle variability of day 3 follicle-stimulating hormone levels and its effect on stimulation quality in in vitro fertilization. Fertility and Sterility, 1990; 54(2):297–302.

24. Khalifa A, Toner JP, Muasher, SJ. Significance of basal follicle-stimulating hormone levels in women with one ovary in a program of in vitro fertilization. Fertility and Sterility, 1992; 57(4):835–839.

25. Nasseri A, Mukherjee T, Grifo JA. Elevated day 3 serum follicle-stimulating hormone and/or estradiol may predict fetal aneuploidy. Fertility and Sterility, 1999; 71(4):715–718.

26. Navot D, Rosenwaks Z, Margalioth EJ. Prognostic assessment of female fecundity. Lancet 1987:2(8560):645–647.

27. Loumaye E, Psalti I, Billion JM et al. Prediction of individual response to controlled ovarian hyperstimulation by means of a clomiphene citrate challenge test. Fertility and Sterility, 1990; 85(3):295–301.

28. Scott RT, Opsahi MS, Leonardi MR et al. Life table analysis of pregnancy rates in a general infertility population relative to ovarian reserve and patient age. Human Reproduction, 1995; 10(7):1706–1710.

29. Scott RT, Leonardi MR, Hofmann GE et al. A prospective evaluation of clomiphene citrate challenge test screening of the general infertility population. Obstetrics and Gynecology, 1993; 82(4 pt. 1):539–544.

30. Sharara FI, Navot D, Beatse SN et al. Cigarette smoking accelerates the development of diminished ovarian reserve as evidenced by the clomiphene citrate challenge test. Fertility and Sterility, 1994; 62(2):257–262.

31. Winslow KL, Oehninger SC, Toner JP et al. The gonadotropin-releasing hormone agonist stimulation test—a sensitive predictor of performance in the flare-up in vitro fertilization cycle. Fertility and Sterility, 1991; 56(4):711–717.

32. Seifer DB, Gardiner AC, Lambert-Messerlian G et al. Day 3 serum inhibin-B is predictive of assisted reproductive technologist outcome. Fertility and Sterility, 1997; 67(1):110–114.

33. Danforth DR, Arbogast LK, Mrough J et al. Dimeric inhibin: A direct marker of ovarian aging. Fertility and Sterility, 1998; 70(1):119–123.

34. Faddy MJ, Gosden RG, Gougeon A et al. Accelerated disappearance of ovarian follicles in mid-life: Implications for forecasting menopause. Human Reproduction, 1992; 7(10):1342–1346.

35. Higgins RV, Van Nagell JR, Woods CH et al. Interobserver variation in ovarian measurements using transvaginal sonography. Gynecologic oncology, 1990; 39(1):69–71.

36. Syrop CH, Willhoite A, Van Voorhis BJ. Ovarian volume: A novel outcome predictor for assisted reproduction. Fertility and Sterility, 1995; 64(6):1167–1171.
37. Lass A, Skull J, McVeigh E. Measurement of ovarian volume by transvaginal sonography before ovulation induction with human menopausal gonadotropin for in vitro fertilization can predictor poor response. Human Reproduction, 1997; 12(2):294–297.
38. Sharara FI, McClamrock HD. The effect of aging on ovarian volume measurements in infertile women. Obstetrics and Gynecology, 1999; 94(1):57–60.
39. Syrop CH, Dawson JD, Husman KJ et al. Ovarian volume may predict assisted reproductive outcomes better than follicle-stimulating hormone concentration on day 3. Human Reproduction, 1999; 14(7):1752–1756.
40. Lass A, Silyr R, Abrams DC et al. Follicular density in ovarian biopsy of infertile women: A novel method to assess ovarian reserve. Human Reproduction 1997; 12(5):1028–1031.
41. Reuss ML, Kline J, Santos R et al. Age and the ovarian follicle pool assessed with transvaginal ultrasonography. American Journal of Obstetrics and Gynecology, 1996; 174(2):624–627.
42. Tomas C, Nuojua-Huttunen S, Martikainen H. Pretreatment transvaginal ultrasound examination predicts ovarian responsiveness to gonadotropins in in-vitro fertilization. Human Reproduction, 1997; 12(2):220–223.
43. Scheffer GJ, Broekmans FJM, Dorland M et al. Antral follicle counts by transvaginal ultrasonography are related to age in women with proven natural fertility. Fertility and Sterility, 1999; 72(5):845–851.
44. Chang MY, Chiang CH, Hsieh TT et al. Use of the antral follicle count to predict the outcome of assisted reproductive technologies. Fertility and Sterility, 1998; 69(3):505–510.
45. Bandsi LFJMM, Broekmans FJM, Eijkemans MJC. Predictors of poor ovarian response in in vitro fertilization: A prospective study comparing basal markers of ovarian reserve. Fertility and Sterility, 2002; 77(2):328–336.

4

Hysterectomy in the Perimenopausal Woman

Frederick W. McLean
Department of Obstetrics and Gynecology, University of Florida College of Medicine, Gainesville, Florida, U.S.A.

Joseph M. Novi
Department of Urogynecology and Reconstructive Pelvic Surgery, Riverside Methodist Hospital, Columbus, Ohio, U.S.A.

I. INTRODUCTION

Hysterectomy remains the most common major gynecologic surgery performed in the United States, with greater than 600,000 procedures performed each year (1). Almost 40% of women in the United States have undergone a hysterectomy by the age of 65 (2). The overall rate of hysterectomy in the United States between 1994 and 1999 was 5.5 per 1000 women, with a low of 0.2 per 1000 in the 15- to 24-year age group, and a high of 11.7 per 1000 in the 40- to 44-year age group, and was essentially unchanged over this time interval. However, hysterectomy rates in perimenopausal women ages 44 to 54 increased significantly, from 8.9 per 1000 in 1994 to 10 per 1000 in 1999 (3). Additionally, women in this perimenopausal age group had the highest percentage of hysterectomies accompanied by bilateral oophorectomy (BSO), with nearly 80% having concomitant BSO at the time of hysterectomy (3). Overall, 71% of concomitant BSO were performed in women whose primary diagnosis was benign (leiomyoma, endometriosis, prolapse) (3).

II. INDICATIONS FOR HYSTERECTOMY

Physicians are now being asked to measure outcomes reflecting not only appropriate care, but also cost-effective care. Insurance companies utilize written guidelines with appropriate indications, as well as prior evaluation and treatment, necessary to grant surgeons permission to proceed with a hysterectomy for a given patient. It is imperative that guidelines are established and adhered to thereby reducing the number of unwarranted surgical procedures.

Few recent publications have looked at guidelines and indications of hysterectomy (4,5). It has been stated that there are more indications for hysterectomy than for any other surgical procedure (6). Rather than applying principles, surgical decision-making, and therapeutic management on the basis of evidence-based guidelines, operative decisions more typically reflect physician values and their previous training and practice patterns. Table 1 lists currently accepted indications for hysterectomy.

A. Uterine Leiomyomas

Uterine leiomyomas (fibroids) are the most common indication for hysterectomy in women of all ages, accounting for approximately one-third of all hysterectomies and almost half of the hysterectomies performed in perimenopausal women in the United States (3,7). Symptoms associated with fibroids include, but are not limited to, abnormal uterine bleeding, pelvic pain, back pain, urinary symptoms (both frequency and incontinence), constipation, repetitive pregnancy loss, dyspareunia, and pelvic pressure (5,8). In the past, fibroids causing enlargement of the uterus approximating a 12-week size gestation was considered an indication for hysterectomy. This size limit has been challenged, and, at this time, surgical intervention for leiomyomas based on uterine size alone in the absence of symptoms is not recommended. If, however, the asymptomatic leiomyoma is of sufficient size and location to cause hydronephrosis, hysterectomy, or myomectomy is indicated (5). In the perimenopausal patient, observation of the asymptomatic leiomyoma not causing hydronephrosis is warranted since the majority of fibroids will regress in size following menopause (9,10). Treatment with GnRH analog therapy is not generally indicated, as the uterus will revert to pre-treatment size within six months of stopping therapy (11). However, some authors have advocated the use of GnRH analogs in women in the late perimenopause with symptomatic fibroids, since this treatment may lead to a rapid progression to menopause following therapy (12).

The presence of a leiomyoma alone is not an indication for surgery. If the patient has abnormal uterine bleeding and leimyoma, other causes of bleeding should be considered. A bleeding lesion of the vulva, vagina, or cervix should be considered. An endometrial biopsy and/or vaginal ultrasound may be necessary to further evaluate the endometrium. Bleeding secondary to uterine fibroids should be a diagnosis of exclusion.

Table 1 Indications for Hysterectomy

Gynecologic Conditions
Uterine Leiomyomas
Endometriosis and Adenomyosis
Genital Prolapse
Dysfunctional/Abnormal Uterine Bleeding
Chronic Pelvic Pain
Pelvic Inflammatory Disease/Tubo-ovarian Abscess
    (ruptured or unresponsive to antibiotic therapy)
Endometrial Hyperplasia/Cancer
Cervical Intraepithelial Neoplasia/Cervical Cancer
Acute Menorraghia (refractory to medical or conservative therapy)

Obstetric Conditions
Uncontrollable Postpartum Hemorrhage
Septic Endometritis with Pyometra

For years it was believed that an enlarging leiomyomata was a threat because of the risk of development of a sarcoma. Many patients had a hysterectomy because their uterus and leiomyoma were increasing in size. In a study in 1996 (Parker), 1300 patients having surgery for leiomyomata had an incidence of sarcoma of 0.23% (13). Although, 371 patients had surgery for what was stated to be "rapidly growing fibroids," only one patient (0.27%) was found to actually have a sarcoma.

B. Endometriosis and Adenomyosis

Endometriosis is the second most common cited indication for hysterectomy in the perimenopausal patient (3). Surgical intervention should be considered when conservative therapy is unsuccessful, when concern exists regarding the long-term consequences of hormone suppression (i.e., osteoporosis), and when the patient no longer desires future fertility. Hysterectomy is indicated when bilateral salpingo-oophorectomy is undertaken and the uterus is determined to be a source of symptoms (14). GnRH analogs have been used effectively to treat endometriosis but their efficacy in treating adenomyosis has not been established.

C. Uterine Prolapse

The third most common cited indication for hysterectomy in the perimenopausal patient is uterine prolapse (3). Symptoms of genital prolapse include pelvic pressure, urinary frequency, urinary hesitancy and retention, detection of a bulge at the introitus, and bleeding secondary to vaginal/cervical erosions. Hysterectomy is indicated when symptoms are present and conservative therapy is unsuccessful or unacceptable for the patient. Currently, there is no data to support the addition of hysterectomy at the time of repair of other pelvic organ prolapse surgery (i.e., relaxation of the anterior and/or posterior vaginal wall) if support of the uterus and vaginal apex is not compromised.

D. Dysfunctional/Abnormal Uterine Bleeding

Control of abnormal bleeding is an indication for approximately 20% of hysterectomies (15). Evaluation of abnormal uterine bleeding is discussed elsewhere in this book (see Chapter 2). Although menorrhagia and the resulting anemia are indications for surgery, the gynecologist must be vigilant in distinguishing between the patient with anemia caused by uterine bleeding and one with bleeding from other sources (i.e., urinary or GI tract, vaginal lesions, etc.) or anemia from metabolic conditions. Hysterectomy is indicated for severe uterine bleeding only when adequate trials of other interventions (medical and/or surgical) have not been effective, or if the patient refuses other interventions. Hysterectomy in the setting of acute, uncontrollable menorrhagia is indicated as a life-saving intervention, though this clinical scenario in the non-pregnant woman is rare.

E. Chronic Pelvic Pain

The patient with chronic pelvic pain should undergo an extensive work-up prior to considering a hysterectomy. The use of hysterectomy to treat idiopathic pelvic pain has not been associated with good success (16). In the patient with pain limited to dysmenorrhea, hysterectomy may provide some relief, though several studies have documented that a significant percentage of these women will have persistent pain following removal of the uterus (17).

F. Pelvic Inflammatory Disease (PID) and Tubo-ovarian Abscess (TOA)

PID is not a common indication for hysterectomy. However, in the patient with ruptured TOA or TOA not responding to conservative therapy, hysterectomy may be considered if future fertility is not desired. Patients with sepsis secondary to pyometra who have failed prior therapy are also candidates for hysterectomy.

G. Endometrial Hyperplasia and Cancer

Endometrial hyperplasia and endometrial cancer together comprise the fourth leading indication for hysterectomy in the perimenopausal patient (3). Rationale for the classification of endometrial hyperplasia as listed in Table 2 is based on the natural history of the disease as shown in long-term follow-up studies (18–20).

Simple hyperplasia carries a very low risk of progression to cancer and can be safely managed with conservative therapy and close follow-up (20). Complex hyperplasia without cytologic atypia may also be managed conservatively (i.e., progestational agents) but does have a risk of progression to cancer that approaches 5% (20). If the patient is unwilling or unable to commit to long-term follow-up, hysterectomy with bilateral salpingo-oophorectomy is indicated.

Tamoxifen was introduced in the United States in 1977 for the treatment of advanced breast cancer. Since that time, the list of indications for its use has expanded. Tamoxifen has been shown to increase the risk of development of endometrial hyperplasia and cancer (21). Because of the high incidence of breast cancer and thus the increased use of Tamoxifen, it is not unusual for the gynecologist to face a situation in which the patient has abnormal uterine bleeding and the transvaginal sonogram shows a marked thickening of the endometrium. Tamoxifen-associated polyps arising in multiple sites in the endometrium have been reported by Schlesinger and Silverberg (21). Endometrial biopsy should be generously used, but the effects of Tamoxifen should be considered when decisions are being made about evaluation and treatment.

Endometrial cancer is the most common gynecologic cancer in the United States and hysterectomy with bilateral salpingo-oophorectomy with intraoperative staging is the preferred initial treatment in the perimenopausal patient. Although adenocarcinoma is the most common cell type, the incidence of other subtypes increases with increasing age (22). In most instances, alternatives to hysterectomy for endometrial cancers should only be considered in rare cases.

Table 2 Classification of Endometrial Hyperplasia

Simple Hyperplasia
Complex Hyperplasia (adenomatous)
Simple Atypical Hyperplasia
Complex Atypical Hyperplasia (adenomatous with atypia)

Source: The World Health Organization.

H. Cervical Intraepithelial Neoplasia (CIN) and Cancer

The treatment of CIN is largely dependent upon the severity, location, and extent of the lesion, as well as the ability of the patient to comply with follow-up (5). Though most cases of CIN I, II, and III can be managed expectantly or with excision or destructive therapy, some instances of CIN III may be treated with hysterectomy if the lesion is large. With the advent of readily available, inexpensive, and accurate HPV subtyping, the indication for hysterectomy may change as more aggressive subtypes warrant more invasive intervention and less aggressive subtypes may be amenable to close observation. Early invasive carcinomas of the cervix currently are best managed with hysterectomy (23).

I. Uncontrollable Postpartum Hemorrhage

Massive postpartum hemorrhage is usually secondary to uterine atony and often responds to aggressive uterotonic therapy. Uterine packing has been advocated by some authors and reports of its successful use have been published (24,25). When conservative therapy is unsuccessful, embolization may be considered in the hemodynamically stable patient. Frequently, however, conservative therapy is unsuccessful and the equipment or personnel needed for embolization is not readily available. Hysterectomy is then warranted as a life-saving intervention. Bleeding secondary to uterine rupture requires laparotomy, while bleeding from uterine inversion is commonly reversed if the inversion can be corrected. Management of persistent bleeding from rupture or inversion should initially be managed with conservative therapy but may ultimately require hysterectomy.

J. Septic Endometritis with Pyometra

Obstetric and gynecologic patients most at risk for sepsis from endometritis or pyometra are those with infected abortions, retained products of conception, tubo-ovarian abscess, and cervical or vaginal cancers. The most common organisms isolated are *Escherichia. coli*, *Klebsiella* and *Enterobacter* species, *Pseudomonas, Proteus,* and *Serratia,* though Clostridial species are particularly virulent. Hysterectomy should be considered if shock persists after uterine curettage and aggressive supportive therapy; if uterine perforation has occurred; if the patient is oliguric; and if the uterus is larger than a 16-week gestation (5). A further indication for hysterectomy includes the presence of clostridial species, though several cases of conservative management in this scenario have been reported (26,27).

III. TYPES OF HYSTERECTOMY

Prior to the advent of antibiotics and advanced surgical technique, the most common type of hysterectomy performed in the early twentieth century was the vaginal hysterectomy (28). By the 1950s, following rapid improvements in anesthesia, suture material, surgical instruments, and surgical technique, the abdominal approach became the preferred route of hysterectomy throughout the United States (28). Currently, abdominal hysterectomy is performed three times as often as vaginal hysterectomy (1). In the 1990s, advances in laparoscopic surgery led its use to facilitate vaginal hysterectomy, though this has had only a small impact on the number of cases performed abdominally (29,30). According to some data, the cost of hysterectomy is two to three times higher than necessary because of the increased use of abdominal and laparoscopic hysterectomy without appropriate guidelines. The evidence-based data, from applying systematic guidelines, strongly suggest that

80% of hysterectomies currently performed can be completed vaginally, taking full advantage of the medical and economic benefits of this surgical route (31–33).

A. Vaginal Hysterectomy

Several recent publications and clinical trials have shown vaginal hysterectomy to be less expensive, carry lower intraoperative and postoperative morbidity, and lead to faster return to normal function when compared to abdominal hysterectomy (31,34–37). In 2001, Varma et al. reported on a five-year project designed to increase the percentage of vaginal hysterectomies performed at their institution, where, at the beginning of the study, 68% were performed abdominally (38). Strict guidelines were introduced, and at the end of the study, 95% of all hysterectomies were performed vaginally. Their findings included a significant decrease in cost, complications, and a significant increase in patient satisfaction. Based on similar data, Kovac (2000) estimated that using these guidelines would result in greater than $1 million saved per 1000 hysterectomies performed (39).

B. Abdominal Hysterectomy

Abdominal hysterectomy remains the procedure of choice for many surgeons. Compared with vaginal hysterectomy, its advantages include better visualization of pelvic anatomy and easier access to adnexal structures. In cases of gynecologic malignancy, an abdominal incision affords access to the upper abdomen which is important for proper staging and optimal tumor debulking. However, the majority of hysterectomies performed abdominally are for benign indications. In the scenario of pelvic organ prolapse, no studies comparing outcomes of abdominal versus vaginal hysterectomy and suspension of the vaginal vault have been published.

C. Laparoscopy

Laparoscopy has quickly become an accepted alternative to laparotomy or vaginal surgery for hysterectomy, cancer staging, and pelvic reconstructive surgery. Initially used as an adjunct to convert abdominal cases to combined laparoscopic/vaginal cases, laparoscopy has frequently been used instead of the standard approaches. Some studies comparing cost, complications, and patient satisfaction have shown laparoscopy to improve outcomes at the expense of increased cost (35,37). Long-term outcomes of laparoscopy compared with laparotomy for pelvic reconstructive surgery have not been reported. Laparoscopy plays an important role in gynecologic cancer, making many previously open surgeries into shorter stay, more cosmetic procedures.

IV. ALTERNATIVES TO HYSTERECTOMY

When faced with a problem that is an indication for hysterectomy, an increasing number of women are interested in alternative therapies. Non-invasive therapies are discussed in detail elsewhere in this book. This section will focus on other surgical treatments for preservation of the uterus.

A. Uterine Artery Embolization (UAE)

UAE was first introduced in the 1990s and has been slowly increasing in popularity. The goal of UAE is the reduction in size of uterine fibroid(s) and consequent reduction in symptoms. McLucas and Adler (2001) reported on 119 consecutive cases of UAE. In their series, 70% of patients had rapid resolution of menorrhagia, pain, and pelvic pressure following UAE (40). At six-months follow-up, the uterine volume decreased an average of 56%. Spies et al. compared 102 patients undergoing UAE to 50 patients having hysterectomy (41). They found a similar rate of patient satisfaction at 6 and 12 months but a significant difference in cost, length of hospitalization, complications, and mean time to return to work favoring the UAE group.

Pain following UAE may persist for two to three weeks following the procedure. Complications occur in approximately 15% of patients, most commonly fever and pain. Failure rate requiring hysterectomy approaches 5%, while life-threatening complications are rare (40). It is estimated that one in 200 women will require emergency hysterectomy due to necrosis leading to uterine abscess and, possibly, septicemia (42). Cases of buttock necrosis, salpingitis, and missed diagnosis of leiomyosarcoma have been reported (42–44).

B. Myomectomy

Although some women are opting for this procedure even when they have completed childbearing, myomectomy, via laparotomy, laparoscopy, or hysteroscopy, has generally been reserved for women with symptomatic fibroids who desire future fertility. In a recent retrospective analysis of reproductive performance before and after abdominal myomectomy, Marchionni et al. found significant increases in conception rate and live birth rate, and a significant decrease in pregnancy loss rate after surgery compared with before surgery (45). Goldberg et al. (2004) compared pregnancy outcomes in women with uterine fibroids after uterine artery embolization versus laparoscopic myomectomy (46). Their findings suggest that pregnancy after UAE is associated with an increased risk for preterm delivery and malpresentation when compared to pregnancy after laparoscopic myomectomy.

When evaluating long-term outcomes after myomectomy compared to UAE, Broder et al. found that at three to five years after the procedure, patients who had undergone UAE were significantly more likely to need additional invasive procedures for the treatment of symptoms than women who had abdominal myomectomy (47).

The chief disadvantage of myomectomy compared to hysterectomy is the risk that new fibroids will form. While myomectomy has been shown to effectively manage symptoms, it does not alter the underlying pathophysiology. Up to 50% of women will have leiomyomas visible on transvaginal ultrasound five years after myomectomy (48). The risk of needing further surgery for symptomatic fibroids ranges from 11% to 26% (49,50). Though hysterectomy is the definitive treatment for fibroids, complications rates from hysterectomy are comparable to those reported after abdominal myomectomy (51,52).

C. Endometrial Ablation

Endometrial ablation procedures became popularized in the late 1980s. Magos et al. introduced transcervical resection of the endometrium (TCRE) into the United Kingdom in 1989 and the procedure became popularized (53). However, after initial enthusiasm, a progressive abandonment developed. This happened because conventional endometrial ablation, by both resection and roller-ball technique, is a highly skill-dependent but underrated procedure. Also, there was poor outcome in patients with uterine pathology; adenomyosis in particular presented a poor outcome. At this time laparoscopic hysterectomy was gaining in popularity and became a real alternative for treatment of dysfunctional bleeding. Complications then began to be reported. There was intraoperative fluid overload, uterine perforation, postoperative bleeding, and even subsequent pregnancy.

McDonald reported a mortality rate of 0.02% following a survey of members of the British Society of Gynaecological Endoscopy in 1992 (54).

Lissak and associates studied the effectiveness and safety of thermal balloon ablation with and without pretreatment of the endometrium (55). Patients with menorrhagia were candidates for treatment with either endometrial ablation or hysterectomy. Two of the patients even had submucosal myomas and six of them had undergone cesarean deliveries in the past. One group consisted of those not treated and another group was treated with a single intramuscular administration of gonadotropin-releasing hormone (GnRH) analog. In the six months of follow-up, there were no significant differences in results between the women treated with immediate or those treated with delayed ablation. This small study suggested that prompt treatment of perimenopausal menorrhagia with thermal balloon ablation is effective and safe. In addition, the GnRH analog endometrial thinning agent is not necessary preoperatively.

The concept of a less skill-dependent ablation of the endometrium was necessary. Some devices such as Novasure and Vestablate deliver electrosurgical energy to the endometrium. Other technologies deliver thermal energy to obtain endometrial destruction. The "Thermachoice®" balloon gained popularity and remains one of the more preferred methods. Recently the cryoablation technique has been developed. A cryoprobe is inserted into the uterine cavity and the temperature is decreased to −80°C (HerOption, Cryogen, San Diego, CA). The advantage of this procedure is that it is not a totally blind procedure and an ultrasound is used for guidance.

In addition, the hydrothermal ablation utilizing circulating heated saline has been evaluated (Hydro Thermablator; BEI Medical Systems: Teterboro, NJ). Saline circulates through the uterus and it is gradually heated to 90°C for 10 minutes, which completely destroys the endometrium. The advantage of the hydrothermal ablation is that the circulating hot saline solution contacts the entire endometrial surface regardless of the size and shape of the uterine cavity.

V. IMMEDIATE AND DELAYED EFFECTS OF HYSTERECTOMY

The most serious complication of any operative procedure is, of course, death. The most common cause of death on a gynecology service is pulmonary embolism. Deep vein thrombosis and pulmonary embolism are major complications that result in significant morbidity and mortality after gynecologic surgery.

There are approximately 260,000 cases annually of clinically diagnosed deep vein thromboses (56). One hundred thousand deaths are attributed to pulmonary embolism annually (57). Deep vein thrombosis has been observed in 14% of patients undergoing gynecologic surgery for benign indications (58). Hormone replacement therapy doubles the risk of venous thromboembolism. Interestingly, the risk is higher near the start of therapy than after long-term care (59).

Surgery predisposes patients to pulmonary embolism, even as late as one month postoperatively. In one study, 25% of the cases of pulmonary embolism occurred between the fifth and the thirtieth postoperative day and 15% were detected more than 30 days postoperatively (60). The incidence of postoperative deep vein thrombosis also has been studied in patients undergoing gynecologic oncology surgery (61). Clarke-Pearson and associates reported on the effects of low-dose heparin and intermittent pneumatic calf compression for the prevention of deep venous thrombosis following gynecologic oncology surgery in a randomized trial (62). Maxwell and associates have concluded that low-molecular-weight heparin and pneumatic compression are similarly effective in the postoperative prophylaxis of thromboembolism (63).

Bergqvist and associates, however, have recently studied 332 patients who were at high risk for venous thromboembolism (64). All patients received enoxaparin (40 mg subcutaneously for 6 to 10 days) and then were randomly assigned to receive either enoxaparin or placebo for another 21 days. The rates of venous thromboembolism were 12.0% in the placebo group and 4.8% in the enoxaparin group. This difference persisted at three months with rates of 13.8% versus 5.5%, respectively. Results of four randomized, prospective, venogram endpoint trials show that LMWH, and possibly unfractioned heparin (UH), given for three to four weeks postoperatively, lower the rate of DVT by about half (65–68). Thus, postoperative gynecologic patients are clearly at risk for deep vein thrombosis. The method of prophylaxis should be determined by the gynecologist, with reference to the particular risk for each patient.

Some have questioned whether hysterectomy offers any protection from future development of nongynecologic cancers. This specific question has been studied in detail, and the figures from the United States as well as a major study conducted in Finland are available for review. In the United States, 550 per 100,000 of all females have had a hysterectomy. One-third of women age 45 years or more have undergone hysterectomy, whereas rates reported in Europe have been lower. In Finland, the rate is 390 per 100,000 women of any age. Their detailed study showed that hysterectomy is not associated with any substantial protective or promoting effect of cancer in general (69).

VI. EFFECT OF HYSTERECTOMY ON PELVIC ORGAN PROLAPSE

Pelvic organ prolapse affects a substantial number of women, with 11% requiring surgical therapy for prolapse in their lifetime (70). Since nearly 40% of women in the United States have undergone a hysterectomy by the age of 65, the effect of hysterectomy on pelvic floor function is of paramount importance (2).

In 1997, Mant et al. explored the epidemiology of genital prolapse in more than 17,000 women aged 25 to 39 years who attended family planning clinics in the United Kingdom between 1968 and 1974 (71). They found that the incidence of prolapse following hysterectomy was 3.6 per 1000 person-years of risk. Also, in their study group, the cumulative risk of prolapse increased from 1% at three years following hysterectomy to 5% 15 years after hysterectomy. Additionally, in this group, the risk of prolapse following hysterectomy was 5.5 times higher in women whose initial hysterectomy was for genital prolapse as opposed to other reasons.

In 1999, Samuelsson et al. reported on the prevalence of pelvic organ prolapse in 487 women aged 20 to 59 years (72). The prevalence of any prolapse in their cohort between the ages of 40 and 49 was 31%, and between ages 50 and 59 was 56%. When compared to women without prior hysterectomy, those women with hysterectomy had a significant increase in their risk for prolapse. Similarly, in a retrospective study of patients undergoing surgery at one urogynecologic center, Moalli et al. found that prior pelvic surgery, including hysterectomy, predisposes women to subsequent pelvic organ prolapse, urinary incontinence, and fecal incontinence compared with controls (73).

In 2002, Hendrix et al. published data from the Women's Health Initiative (74). They concluded that prior hysterectomy was not associated with an increased risk of prolapse. However, the authors state that the pelvic examination was performed only in the supine position, which has been shown to underestimate prolapse compared with examination in a birthing chair at a 45° angle (75). Also, neither a split speculum examination nor the Pelvic Organ Prolapse Quantification (POP-Q) system were employed, introducing the possibility of underreporting of prolapse.

Based on available data, it is our belief that the cumulative risk of pelvic organ prolapse increases in a linear fashion over time following hysterectomy. We recommend several steps to decrease the likelihood of vaginal vault prolapse following hysterectomy. First, whether operating from the vaginal or abdominal approach, an effort should be made to incorporate the cardinal-uterosacral complex into the vaginal apex after removal of the urterus. The efficacy of this procedure has recently been demonstrated (76). Second, preoperative examinations should include the supine, 45° angle and/or standing positions to more accurately identify prolapse. The identification of prolapse prior to surgery should aid in surgical planning to address the prolapse intraoperatively. Finally, if the hysterectomy is undertaken for uterine prolapse, consideration should be given to adding a vaginal vault suspension to the surgical plan, recognizing that vaginal vault prolapse frequently accompanies uterine prolapse.

VII. PSYCHOLOGICAL EFFECTS OF HYSTERECTOMY

The psychological outcomes of hysterectomy and oophorectomy for nonmalignant indications have been studied in a meta-analysis (77). The majority of retrospective studies show an adverse psychological outcome after hysterectomy. However, all prospective studies show that the incidence of depressed mood is higher before hysterectomy owing to the pre-existing psychiatric illness and psychosocial problems as manifested by gynecologic symptoms. The therapeutic effects of hysterectomy, with or without oophorectomy, may include improvement of mood in some but not all patients where proper case selection, psychiatric evaluation, and preoperative counseling are arranged. Psychological symptoms actually improve in the majority of women with the relief of distressing gynecologic symptoms and the correction of ovarian hormone deficiency, but hysterectomy with or without salpingo-oophorectomy may not be of any benefit in women with prior psychiatric illness or in those with personality and psychosocial problems.

The incidence of depressed mood is high in women before hysterectomy. This finding is usually based on the effects of prolonged heavy periods, chronic pelvic pain, and severe premenstrual symptoms that warrant surgical treatment. Khastgir and associates reported on their study of psychological outcomes and noted that in women with pre-existing psychiatric illness, the therapeutic effect of hysterectomy, with or without oophorectomy, included both the cure of physical symptoms and the improvement of mood (77). However, in women with predisposing personality problems, depressed mood may persist or grow with the distress of hysterectomy.

Ovarian hormone deficiency from hysterectomy alone may be responsible for the negative effect on mood and, without routine endocrinologic monitoring, any indicated estrogen replacement following hysterectomy may be missed. Estrogen plus testosterone replacement following hysterectomy with or without bilateral oophorectomy has been shown to reduce the incidence of the depressed state. The practice of regular endocrinologic and clinical monitoring following hysterectomy to detect the need for estrogen or combined estrogen-testosterone replacement following bilateral oophorectomy may be considered to reduce the incidence of posthysterectomy depression.

VIII. EFFECT OF HYSTERECTOMY ON SEXUAL FUNCTION

Several studies have attempted to evaluate the effect of hysterectomy on sexual function (78–84). The results have been mixed, with some showing a negative effect, some demonstrating no effect, and some showing an improvement in sexual function. As recently as 2003, a literature review of sexual function and hysterectomy by Maas et al. concluded the "prehysterectomy sexual functioning and psychological state are significant predictors for posthysterectomy sexual dysfunction ..." (80). The authors further stated that "a minority of women report developing sexual dysfunctions as a result of hysterectomy."

Roovers et al. performed a prospective observational study of 413 women undergoing hysterectomy in the Netherlands (85). Patients included in the study were scheduled for vaginal hysterectomy, total abdominal hysterectomy, or subtotal abdominal hysterectomy, with the surgical approach decided upon by the patient and the individual surgeon. Though this was not a randomized trial, the patients were similar in age, parity, body mass index, preoperative frequency of sexual activity, bothersome sexual problems before surgery, and duration of relationship with their partner. Patients were administered a validated questionnaire prior to surgery and six months after surgery. The authors concluded that "sexual wellbeing improves after vaginal hysterectomy, subtotal abdominal hysterectomy, and total abdominal hysterectomy. The type of technique does not seem to determine the persistence or development of bothersome problems during sexual activity." A similar study by Roussis et al. in 2004 found comparable results (78).

In 2004, Dragisic and Milad prospectively evaluated sexual function and patient expectations of sexual function before and after hysterectomy (79). Seventy-five patients completed validated questionnaires at the time of their hysterectomy and six months after surgery. The majority of patients underwent abdominal hysterectomy (56%), with uterine fibroids as the most common indication for surgery (80%). The authors found that "most patients expected and experienced no change in sexual desire, orgasm frequency, or orgasm intensity." Additionally, patients were significantly less likely to complain of pain with intercourse after the procedure (8.1%) as compared with before the procedure (43%, p <0.001). 82% of patients who reported pelvic pain as the primary indication for surgery noted decreased pain after surgery.

IX. OOPHORECTOMY

The decision to perform oophorectomy in the perimenopausal woman at the time of hysterectomy for benign disease is controversial. While some studies have estimated that prophylactic oophorectomy at the time of hysterectomy would result in a 5% reduction in the subsequent development of ovarian cancer, these studies are based on retrospective analyses of women who developed ovarian cancer after hysterectomy (86–89). A similar trial by Charoenkwan et al. in Thailand reported that only 13 (1.73%) of 752 women with epithelial ovarian cancer had undergone a hysterectomy prior to the diagnosis of ovarian cancer (90). The authors concluded that based on their findings, prophylactic oophorectomy at the time of hysterectomy for benign disease should not be recommended. Additionally, they found that routine oophorectomy for women over age 45 undergoing hysterectomy would result in only a 0.16% reduction in the annual incidence of ovarian cancer.

The data to support prophylactic oophorectomy at the time of hysterectomy in women with a BRCA1 or BRCA2 germline mutation is more compelling. Olivier et al., in 2004, performed a retrospective review of 128 women with BRCA1, BRCA2, or who belonged to a Heredity Breast/Ovarian Cancer (HBOC) family who had prophylactic oophorectomy or salpingo-oophorectomy performed (91). Among the 38 women with oophorectomy only, no occult carcinomas were identified. However, three (8%) developed papillary serous carcinoma of the peritoneum during the 45 months of follow-up.

Among the 90 patients who had salpingo-oophorectomy, five (5.6%) were found to have occult carcinoma apparent only on microscopic examination. These included two fallopian tube carcinomas, two ovarian carcinomas, and one fallopian tube/ovarian carcinoma. Of the 90 women who had salpingo-oophorectomy, none developed papillary serous carcinoma of the peritoneum during follow-up.

In 2000, Matloff et al. conducted a survey of the National Society of Genetic Counsellors (NSGC) Special Interest Group (SIG) in Cancer (92). Given the hypothetical scenario of personal genetic testing showing a BRCA1 or BRCA2 mutation at age 35, 25% reported that they would undergo prophylactic bilateral mastectomies and 68% would have prophylactic bilateral oophorectomy. If they tested positive for a hereditary nonpolyposis colon cancer (HNPCC) mutation, 17% would elect prophylactic colectomy, 54% prophylactic hysterectomy, and 52% prophylactic oophorectomy. Interestingly, 68% would not bill their insurance companies for the genetic testing for fear of discrimination.

While it is not cost-effective to screen the general population for genetic mutations, screening of high-risk groups is appropriate. If a woman is found to have a BRCA1, BRCA2, or HNPCC mutation, recommendations for surveillance for ovarian cancer include semiannual or annual transvaginal ultrasound and testing for CA-125 levels beginning between the ages of 25 and 35 years (92). Unfortunately, the effectiveness of detecting ovarian cancers at earlier and more treatable stages using thiese recommendations has not been demonstrated.

At the present time, consideration of oophorectomy at the time of hysterectomy for benign indications in the perimenopausal woman should take into account the patient's wishes, her family history, and the clinical scenario. If the family history suggests the possibility of a genetic mutation at high risk for ovarian cancer, a referral to a genetic counselor for testing should be made. If the patient carries a germline mutation, strong consideration should be given to performing bilateral oophorectomy. Furthermore, if the procedure planned is a vaginal hysterectomy, the addition of laparoscopy to insure the removal of all ovarian and fallopian tube tissue should be considered. In the patient who does not carry a genetic cancer mutation, the role of ovarian hormones in the maintenance of sexual function, bone health, and cardiovascular health should be discussed.

X. SUMMARY

Hysterectomy continues to be the most common major gynecologic surgery performed in the United States each year. By age 65, nearly 40% of women have undergone hysterectomy for a variety of indications. Depending upon the clinical scenario, a number of therapeutic options are available for the woman who wants to retain her uterus. Preoperative counseling in the woman who is considering hysterectomy should include the disposition of the ovaries, and the potential impact that the surgery may have on pelvic floor function.

REFERENCES

1. Matloff ET, Shappell H, Brierly K et al. What would you do? Specialists' perspectives on cancer genetic testing, prophylactic surgery, and insurance discrimination. J Clin Oncol 2000; 18:2484–2492.
2. Olivier RI, van Beurden M, Lubsen MAC et al. Clinical outcome of prophylactic oophorectomy in BRCA1/BRCA2 mutation carriers and events during follow-up. Br J Cancer 2004; 90:1492–1497.

3. Maas CP, Weijenborg PT, ter Kuile MM. The effect of hysterectomy on sexual functioning. Ann Rev Sex Res 2003; 14:83–113.

4. Dragisic KG, Milad MP. Sexual functioning and patient expectations of sexual functioning after hysterectomy. Am J Obstet Gynecol 2004; 190:1416–1418.

5. Roovers JW, van der Bom JG, van der Vaart CH et al. Hysterectomy and sexual well-being: prospective observational study of vaginal hysterectomy, subtotal abdominal hysterectomy, and total abdominal hysterectomy. BMJ 2003; 327:774–779.

6. Carlson KJ, Nichols DH, Schiff I. Indications for hysterectomy. NEJM 1993; 328:856–860.

7. Farquhar CM, Steiner CA. Hysterectomy rates in the United States 1990–1997. Obstet Gynecol 2002; 99:229–234.

8. Kovac SR. Clinical opinion: Guidelines for hysterectomy. Am J Obstet Gynecol 2004; 191:635–640.

9. Keshavarz H, Hillis SD, Kieke BA et al. Hysterectomy surveillance—United States 1994–1999. MMWR 2002; 51:1–8.

10. Lefebrve G, Allaire C, Jeffrey J et al. Hysterectomy: SOGC clinical practice guidelines. J Obstet Gynaecol Can 2002; 109:1–12.

11. Kovac SR. Decision-directed hysterectomy: A possible approach to improve medical and economic outcomes. Int J Obstet Gynecol 2000; 71:156–159.

12. Kovac SR, Cruikshank SH, Retto HF. Laparoscopy-assisted vaginal hysterectomy. J Gynecol Surg 1990 Fall; 6(3):185–93.

13. Morley GW. Indications for hysterectomy. In Thompson JD, Rock JA, eds: TeLinde's Operative Gynecology: Update. Philadelphia, JB Lippincott; 1993, pp 1–11.

14. Queileu V, Cosson M, Paramentier D et al. The impact of laparoscopic surgery on vaginal hysterectomy. Gynecol Endosc 1993; 2:89–91.

15. Cosson M, Subtil D, Switala I et al. The feasibility of vaginal hysterectomy. Eur J Obstet Gynecol 1996; 64:95–99.

16. Schlesinger C, Silverberg SG. Tamoxifen-associated polyps (basalomas) arising in multiple endometriotic foci: A case report and review of the literature. Gynecol Oncol 1999 May; 73(2):305–311.

17. Parker WH, Fu YS, Berek JS. Uterine sarcoma in patients operated on for presumed leiomyoma and rapidly growing leiomyoma. Obstet Gynecol 1996; 83:414–418.

18. Baak JP, Wisse-Brekelmans EC, Fleege JC et al. Assessment of the risks of endometrial cancer and hyperplasia by means of morphologic and morphometric features. Pathol Res Pract 1992; 188:856–859.

19. Ferenczy A, Gelfand M. The biologic significance of cytologic atypia in progestogen-treated endometrial hyperplasia. Am J Obstet Gynecol 1989; 160:126–131.

20. Kurman RJ, Kaminski PF, Norris HJ. The behavior of endometrial hyperplasia. A long-term study of "untreated" hyperplasia in 170 patients. Cancer 1985; 56:403–412.

21. Clagett GP, Reisch JS. Prevention of venous thromboembolism in general surgical patients. Results of meta-analysis. Ann Surg 1988; 208:227–240.

22. Dalen JE, Alpert JS. Natural history of pulmonary embolism. Prog Cardiovasc Dis 1975; 17:257–270.

23. Walsh JJ, Bonnar J, Wright FW. A study of pulmonary embolism and deep leg thrombosis after major gynaecological surgery using labelled fibrinogen-phlebography and lung scanning. J Obstet Gynaecol Br Commonw 1974; 81:311–316.

24. Vandenbroucke JP, Helmerhorst FM. Risk of venous thrombosis with hormone replacement therapy. Lancet 1996 Oct 12; 348(9033):972.

25. Bergqvist D, Lindblad B. A 30-year survey of pulmonary embolism verified at autopsy: An analysis of 1274 surgical patients. Br J Surg 1985 Feb; 72(2):105–108.

26. Crandon AJ, Knotts J. Incidence of postoperative deep vein thrombosis in gynaecological oncology. Aust NZ J Obstet Gynecol 1983; 23:216–219.

27. Clarke-Pearson DL, Synan IS, Dodge R et al. A randomized trial of low-dose heparin at the intermittent pneumatic calf compression for the prevention of deep venous thrombosis following gynecologic oncology surgery. Am J Obstet Gynecol 1993;168:1146–1153.

28. Maxwell GL, Synan I, Dodge R et al. Pneumatic compression versus low molecular weight heparin in gynecologic oncology surgery: A randomized trial. Obstet Gynecol 2001 Dec; 98(6):989–995.

29. Bergqvist D, Lowe GD, Berstad A et al. Prevention of venous thromboembolism after surgery: A review of enoxaparin. Br J Surg 1992 Jun; 79(6):495–498.

30. Bergqvist D, Benoni G, Bjorgel O, et al. Extending enoxaparin 1 month after hospital discharge reduced thromboembolism after elective hip surgery. N Engl J Med 1996; 335:696–700.

31. Planes A, Vochelle N, Darmon J-Y et al. Risk of deep-venous thrombosis after hospital discharge in patients having undergone total hip replacement; Double-blind randomised comparison of enoxaparin versus placebo. Lancet 1996; 348:224–228.

32. Manganelli D, Pazzagli M, Mazzantini D. Prolonged prophylaxis with unfractioned heparin is effective to reduce delayed deep vein thrombosis in total hip replacement. Respiration 1998; 65(5):369–374.

33. Dahl OE, Andreassen G, Aspelin T et al. Prolonged thromboprophylaxis following hip replacement surgery—results of a double-blind, prospective, randomized, placebo-controlled study with dalteparin (Fragmin). Thromb Haemost 1997; 77:26–31.

34. Luoto R, Auvinen A, Pukkala E et al. Hysterectomy and subsequent risk of cancer. Int J Epidemiol 1997 June; 26(3):476–483.

35. Khastgir G, Studd JW, Catalan J. The psychological outcome of hysterectomy. Gynecol Endocrinol 2000 April; 14(2):132–141.

36. Magos AL, Baumann R, Turnbull AC. Transcervical resection of endometrium in women with menorrhagia. BMJ 1989 May 6; 298(6682):1209–1212.

37. McDonald R, Phipps J, Singer A. Endometrial ablation: A safe procedure. Gynaecol Endosc 1992; 1:7–9.

38. Lissak A, Fruchter O, Mashiach S et al. Immediate versus delayed treatment of perimenopausal bleeding due to benign cancer by balloon thermal ablation. J Am Assoc Gynecol Laparosc 1999 May; 6(2):145–150.

39. Goldberg J, Burd I, Price FV et al. Leiomyosarcoma in a premenopausal patient after uterine artery embolization. Am J Obstet Gynecol 2004; 191(5):1733–1735.

40. Porcu G, Roger V, Jacquier A et al. Uterus and bladder necrosis after uterine artery embolization for postpartum haemorrhage. BJOG 2005; 112(1):122–123.

41. Rajan DK, Beecroft JR, Clark TW et al. Risk of intrauterine infectious complications after uterine artery embolization. J Vasc Radiol 2004; 15(12):1415–1421.

42. Spies JB, Cooper JM, Worthinton-Kirsch R et al. Outcome of uterine artery embolization and hysterectomy for leiomyomas: Results of a multicenter study. Obstet Gynecol Surv 2004; 59(12):819–820.

43. McLucas B, Adler L. Uterine fibroid embolization compared with myomectomy. Int J Gynaecol Obstet 2001; 74:297–299.

44. Sculpher M, Manca A, Abbott J et al. Cost effectiveness analysis of laparoscopic hysterectomy compared with standard hysterectomy: Results from a randomized trial. BMJ 2004; 328:132–134.

45. Miskry T, Magos A. Randomized, propective, double-blind comparison of abdominal and vaginal hysterectomy in women without uterovaginal prolapse. Acta Obstet Gynecol Scand 2003; 82:351–358.

46. Ribiero SC, Ribiero RM, Santos NC. A randomized study of total abdominal, vaginal and laparoscopic hysterectomy. Int J Gynaecol Obstet 2003; 83(1):37–43.

47. Taylor SM, Romero AA, Kammerer-Doak DN. Abdominal hysterectomy for the enlarged myomatous uterus compared with vaginal hysterectomy with morcellation. Am J Obstet Gynecol 2003; 189(6):1579–1582.

48. Kovac SR. Similar outcomes in patients with similar indications. Obstet Gynecol 2000; 95(6):787–793.

49. Varma R, Tahseen S, Lokugamage AU et al. Vaginal route as the norm when planning hysterectomy for benign conditions: Change in practice. Obstet Gyencol 2001; 97:613–616.

50. Lethaby A, Vollenhoven B, Sowter M. Efficacy of pre-operative gonadotropin hormone releasing analogues for women with uterine fibroids undergoing hysterectomy or myomectomy: A systematic review. Br J Obstet Gynaecol 2002; 109:1097–1108.

51. Sam C, Hamid MA, Swan N. Pyometra associated with retained products of conception. Obstet Gynecol 1999; 93:840.

52. Lichtenberg ES, Henning C. Conservative management of clostridial endometritis. Am J Obstet Gynecol 2004; 191:266–270.

53. Chung MK. Interstitial cystitis in persistent posthysterectomy chronic pelvic pain. JSLS 2004; 8(4):329–333.

54. Stovall TG, Ling FW, Crawford DA. Hysterectomy for chronic pelvic pain of presumed uterine etiology. Obstet Gynecol 1990; 75:676–679.

55. Lee NC, Dicker RC, Rubin GL. Confirmation of the preoperative diagnoses for hysterectomy. Am J Obstet Gynecol 1984; 150:283–287.

56. Goodwin SC, Wong GC. Uterine artery embolization for uterine fibroids: A radiologist's perspective. Clin Obstet Gynecol 2001; 44(2):412–424.

57. Guarnaccia MM, Rein MS. Traditional surgical approaches to uterine fibroids: Abdominal myomectomy and hysterectomy. Clin Obstet Gynecol 2001; 44(2):385–400.

58. Kjerulff KH, Erickson BA, Langenberg PW. Chronic gynecological conditions reported by US women: Findings from the National Health Interview Survey, 1984 to 1992. Am J Public Health 1996; 86(2):195–199.

59. Lepine LA, Hillis SD, Marchbanks PA. Hysterectomy surveillance—United States, 1980–1993. MMWR 1997; 178:977–981.

60. Weir E. The public health toll of endometriosis. CMAJ 2001; 164(8):1201.

61. Shoupe D. Hysterectomy or an alternative? Hosp Pract 2000; 35(9):55–62.

62. Thompson JD. Hysterectomy. In: Thompson JD, Rock JA, eds. Te Linde's Operative Gynecology, 7th edition. Philadelphia: JB Lippincott, 1992, 684.

63. Olsen AL, Smith VJ, Bergstrom JO et al. Epidemiology of surgically managed pelvic organ prolapse and urinary incontinence. Obstet Gynecol 1997; 89:501–506.

64. Roussis NP, Waltrous L, Kerr A et al. Sexual reponse in the patient after hysterectomy: Total abdominal versus supracervical versus vaginal procedure. Am J Obstet Gynecol 2004; 190:1427–1428.

65. Gutl P, Greimel ER, Roth R et al. Women's sexual behavior, body image and satisfaction with surgical outcomes after hysterectomy: A comparison of vaginal and abdominal surgery. J Pschosom Obstet Gynaecol 2002; 23:51–59.

66. Weber AM, Walters MD, Schover LR et al. Functional outcomes and satisfaction after abdominal hysterectomy. Am J Obstet Gynecol 1999; 181:530–535.

67. Zussman L, Zussman S, Sunley R. Sexual response after hysterectomy-oophorectomy: Recent studies and reconsideration of psychogenesis. Am J Obstet Gynecol 1981; 140:725–728.

68. Bellerose SB, Binik YM. Body image and sexuality in oophorectomized women. Arch Sexual Behav 1993; 22:435–439.

69. Fedele L, Parazzini F, Luchini L et al. Recurrence of fibroids after myomectomy: A trans vaginal ultrasound study. Hum Reprod 1995; 10:1795–1796.

70. Malone LJ. Myomectomy: Recurrence after removal of solitary and multiple myomas. Obstet Gynecol 1969; 34:200–203.

71. Acien P, Quereda F. Abdominal myomectomy: Results of a simple operative technique. Fertil Steril 1996; 65:41–51.

72. LaMorte AI, Lalwani S, Diamond MP. Morbidity associated with abdominal myomectomy. Obstet Gynecol 1993; 82(6):897–900.

73. Hillis SD, Marchbanks PA, Peterson HB. Uterine size and risk of complications among women undergoing abdominal hysterectomy for leiomyomas. Obstet Gynecol 1996; 87(4):539–543.

74. Broder MS, Goodwin S, Chen G. Comparison of long-term outcomes of myomectomy and uterine artery embolization. Obstet Gynecol 2002; 100(5):864–868.

75. Goldberg J, Pereira L, Berghella V et al. Pregnancy outcomes after treatment for fibromyomata: Uterine artery embolization versus laparoscopic myomectomy. Am J Obstet Gynecol 2004; 191(1):18–21.

76. Marchionni M, Fambrini M, Zambelli V et al. Reproductive performance before and after abdominal myomectomy: A retrospective analysis. Fertil Steril 2004; 82(1):154–159.

77. Charoenkwan K, Srisomboon J, Suprasert P. Role of prophylactic oophorectomy at the time of hysterectomy in ovarian cancer prevention in Thailand. J Obstet Gynaecol Res 2004; 30(2):20–23.

78. Golan A. GnRH analogues in the treatment of uterine fibroids. Hum Reprod 1996; 11:33–41.

79. ACOG Women's Health Physicians. Ovarian, endometrial, and colorectal cancers. Obstet Gynecol 2004; 104:77S–84S.

80. Pecorelli S, Angioli R, Favalli G. Systemic therapy for gynecologic neoplasms: Ovary, cervix and endometrium. Cancer Chemother Biol Response Modif 2003; 21:565–584.

81. Bagga R, Jain V, Kalra J. Uterovaginal packing with rolled gauze in postpartum hemorrhage. Med Gen Med 2004; 6(1):50.

82. Baskett TF. J Obstet Gynaecol Can 2004; 26(9):805–808.

83. Mant J, Painter R, Vessey M. Epidemiology of genital prolapse: Observations from the Oxford Family Palnning Association Study. Br J Obstet Gynaecol 1997; 104(5):579–585.

84. Samuelsson EC, Victor FT, Tibblin G et al. Signs of genital prolapse in a Swedish population of women 20 to 59 years of age and possible related factors. Am J Obstet Gynecol 1999; 180(2):1415–1423.

85. Moalli PA, Ivy SJ, Meyn LA et al. Risk factors associated with pelvic floor disorders in women undergoing surgical repair. Obstet Gynecol 2003; 101:869–874.

86. Hendrix SL, Clark A, Nygaard I et al. Pelvic organ prolapse in the Women's Health Initiative: Gravity and gravidity. Am J Obstet Gynecol 2002; 186:1160–1166.

87. Barber MD, Lambers AR, Visco AG et al. Effect of patient position on clinical evaluation of pelvic organ prolapse. Obstet Gynecol 2000; 96:18–22.

88. Montella JM, Morrill MY. Effectiveness of the McCall culdoplasty in maintaining support after vaginal hysterectomy. Int Urogynecol J Pelvic Floor Dysfunct 2004; 15(6):24–29.

89. Das N, Kay VJ, Mahmood TA. Current knowledge of risks and benefits of prophylactic oophorectomy at hysterectomy for benign disease in United Kingdom and Republic of Ireland. Eur J Obstet Gynecol Reprod Biol 2003; 109:76–79.

90. Sightler SE, Boike GM, Estape RE et al. Ovarian cancer in women with prior hysterectomy. Obstet Gynecol 1991; 78:681–684.

91. Averette HE, Nguyen HN. The role of prophylactic oophorectomy in cancer prevention. Gynecol Oncol 1994; 55:S38–41.

92. McGowan L. Ovarian cancer after hysterectomy. Obstet Gynecol 1987; 69:386–389.

5

Obstetrical Issues in Women of Advanced Reproductive Age

Douglas S. Richards
Department of Obstetrics and Gynecology, University of Florida College of Medicine, Gainesville, Florida, U.S.A.

I. INTRODUCTION

Increasing numbers of women are having children in their later reproductive years. This chapter will outline the changing demographics in the "older gravida" and discuss pregnancy issues unique to this group. While there are numerous pregnancy complications that have historically been associated with advancing maternal age, we will see that many of them have minimal impact if an older woman is healthy. If a pre-pregnancy evaluation shows the absence of complicating factors a mature woman can be optimistic about the likelihood of a good pregnancy outcome.

II. DEMOGRAPHICS

The birth rate (births per 1000 women) of women in the older age ranges fell precipitously from 1960 until about 1977 (1). As shown in Figure 1, the rate fell by 66% in women aged 35 to 39 and by 81% of women aged 40 to 44. This fall undoubtedly was due to the more widespread availability of reliable contraceptives, and changes in the desired number of children. However, starting in 1977, the birth rate trend in women over age 35 reversed, and by 1999 had rebounded to 69% of the 1960 rate for women aged 35 to 39 and to 47% of the 1960 rate in the 40- to 44-year-old bracket.

This reversal is not due to a return to the large families of the 1960s, but rather is a result of women who reached childbearing age in the 70s and 80s delaying the birth of their first child. Figure 2 shows the change in birth orders of children born to women aged 35 to 39 over the last four decades. While in 1960, 65% of women giving birth in this age bracket had already had three or more children, this figure fell to 29% in 1979 and 10% in 2000 (2,3). Conversely, only 17% of these women in 1960 were having their first

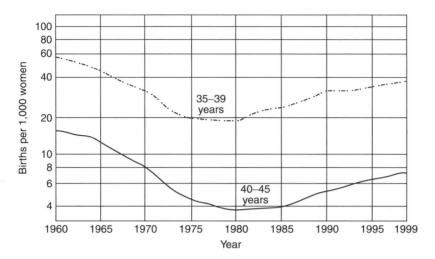

Figure 1 Birth rate trends for older women from 1960 to 1999. Note that the y-axis is a logarithmic scale.

or second child compared to 55% in the year 2000. Census Bureau statistics show that in 2000, among women aged 35 to 39 years old, 20% had not had any children, while in 1976, this figure was only 10%. Figures from the 2000 census show that 19% of women aged 40 to 44 were childless (4).

Reasons that women are delaying childbearing are not completely established. Certainly, both the availability of contraceptives and the trend toward later marriage play a part. Nowadays many women have access to careers that are financially and personally satisfying. Many are reluctant to take time off from work in the early stages of their careers in order to bear and care for children.

Because of the demographic factors outlined above, the birth rate in women over age 35 has increased dramatically in the past two decades. Even more impressive than the

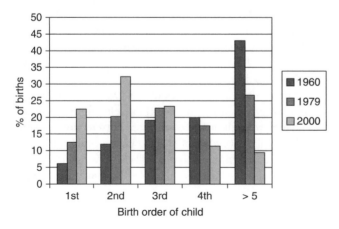

Figure 2 Birth order of children born to women aged 35 to 39 in three representative years.

increased birth rate is the increased total number of children born to women in the older age categories. For example, the number of births in the United States to women aged 35 to 39 increased by 335% between 1979 and 2000 (from 135,096 to 452,057) (4). While this is partially explained by the higher birth rate described earlier, it is largely a reflection of the large number of women of the post-World War II "baby boom" who are moving into these age brackets.

III. CHROMOSOMAL ABNORMALITIES

A. Genetic Counseling

It is well established that as a woman ages there is an increased risk of aneuploidy in her offspring. Age-associated dysfunction of the spindle apparatus during meiosis can cause non-disjuction resulting in aneuploidy in the oocyte. The risk that a resulting fetus will have an abnormal karyotype is one of the most easily quantifiable risks of childbearing at an increased age. Since reliable statistics are available (5) (Fig. 3) counseling regarding the magnitude of these risk is relatively straightforward. While trisomy 21 is the most common aneuploidy in live born infants, and thus garners the most attention among the lay public, it is important for providers to discuss with patients other aneuploidies such as trisomy 18 and 13, and those involving the sex chromosomes.

It is currently the standard of care to offer invasive testing for genetic diagnosis to all women who will be 35 or older at the time of delivery. Age 35 became the traditional time at which to offer amniocentesis because this is the age at which the chance of an abnormal result is roughly equivalent to the risk of a complication from amniocentesis (1 in 200). As Figure 3 shows, there is an accelerating increase in the risk of an abnormal karyotype after this age.

All women of increased age should be given the opportunity to have genetic counseling regarding testing options. This is best done by a genetic counselor who can

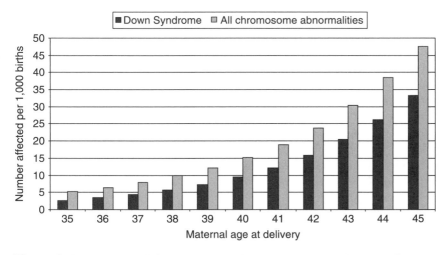

Figure 3 Chance that an infant will have a chromosome abnormality depending on the mother's age at delivery.

evaluate the family history and other factors affecting the risk of genetic disease in the fetus. For example, while the main concern of an older woman may be the risk of Down syndrome, a genetic history may uncover a family history of cystic fibrosis. The counselor could arrange genetic testing for this condition as well.

Counseling regarding testing for genetic disease in the fetus is usually non-directive in nature. Given the tremendous diversity among patients concerning the acceptability of abortion, willingness to accept the risks of invasive procedures, and desires for definitive answers regarding the genetic makeup of the fetus, there is no "right" course of action. The counselor should gather information from a patient regarding genetic risks, provide information about available tests, and help couples explore their feelings about the appropriateness of these tests.

B. Invasive Genetic Testing

Amniocentesis is the time-honored procedure for determining the fetal karyotype. This involves introducing a thin-gauge needle through the uterine wall into the amniotic cavity under direct ultrasound guidance. About 20 ml of amniotic fluid is withdrawn and this fluid is sent to a cytogenetics laboratory for processing. A culture of amniocytes is established and in 10 to 14 days multiple cells can be analyzed for karyotype. Missing or extra chromosomes, translocations, and chromosome deletions and dysmorphisms are all uncovered with this technique.

Genetic amniocentesis is usually performed between 15 and 18 weeks gestation. There is no upper limit beyond which the test can be performed, but there is generally no advantage in terms of safety or ease of performing the procedure after 18 weeks. The upper legal limit for pregnancy termination in most states is 24 weeks gestation, so if this option is to be available, amniocentesis must be done by 22 weeks. Of course, most patients would like results as soon as they can safely be obtained. Because techniques for ultrasound guidance have improved, it is now technically possible to perform amniocentesis as early as 11 weeks gestation. However, a large, prospective, randomized study showed that amniocentesis before 15 weeks gestation results in more pregnancy losses, an increased incidence of fluid leakage, a higher rate of unsuccessful procedures, increased numbers with failed amniocyte culture, and an increased incidence of clubbed foot in the baby (6).

It has been shown that the complication rate from genetic amniocentesis is lowest when the procedure is performed by a physician who performs it frequently (7). In most cases, obstetricians refer patients for genetic counseling and Maternal Fetal Medicine specialists who work at established prenatal diagnosis centers. Advantages of this specialized approach include the availability of a genetic counselor for pre-procedure counseling, the increased safety by having the amniocentesis performed by a practiced individual, the proper handling of specimens, the prompt communication to the patient of results, and the availability of counseling regarding the significance of abnormal results.

A major concern of women considering amniocentesis is the possibility of complications. In spite of technical advances that have made amniocentesis easier, with a lower rate of bloody taps and need for repeat procedures, losses attributable to amniocentesis can occur. The most common complication obviously attributable to the procedure is immediate onset of fluid leakage. Fortunately, with bed rest, most cases reseal spontaneously, and the pregnancy is continued. Other rare complications include infection, fetal death, abruption, and preterm labor. The risk of pregnancy loss attributable to genetic amniocentesis at the "standard" time is generally considered to be 0.5%, or one loss per 200 procedures (8).

Amniocentesis results are typically not available to a patient until 17 to 20 weeks gestation. By that time, family and acquaintances are usually aware of the pregnancy and fetal movement may be perceived, increasing the psychologic distress of pregnancy termination. For this reason, and because of the increased medical risks of mid-second trimester abortion, there has been interest in developing first trimester genetic testing. Chorionic villus sampling (CVS), in which a needle or catheter is passed into the villi of the developing placenta at about 10 to 12 weeks gestation, came into widespread use in the 1980s. The first method of performing CVS to gain acceptance was the transcervical approach. With this technique, the woman is placed on the exam table in a lithotomy position and a speculum is placed in the vagina to visualize the cervix. After cleansing the cervix, a catheter is guided with the aid of transabdominal ultrasound through the cervix into the placenta. Once the catheter is in place, suction is applied to aspirate fragments of villi from the placenta. In the 1990s a transabdominal approach to CVS was developed. With this procedure, a needle (usually 19 or 20 gauge) is placed through the maternal abdominal wall and uterine wall into the placenta under ultrasound guidance for aspiration of villi. The villi are then sent to the cytogenics laboratory for culture, and a karyotype is obtained in 10 to 14 days.

Most studies have shown that CVS is associated with a higher pregnancy loss rate than amniocentesis (9). The total pregnancy loss rate after CVS is about 5% but most losses are not directly attributable to the procedure. CVS is done early enough in pregnancy that spontaneous abortion from causes unrelated to the invasive testing are still relatively common. In contrast, spontaneous losses are rare after 15 weeks, the time at which amniocentesis is usually performed. Because many chromosomally abnormal fetuses that are alive at 10 weeks will have died spontaneously by 15 weeks, chromosome testing by CVS in the first trimester yields a higher rate of abnormalities than testing with amniocentesis in the second trimester. Therefore, CVS has a higher "loss rate" from induced abortions of abnormal fetuses. Even taking into account these factors, there seems to be a higher procedure related loss rate from CVS (1% to 2%) than amniocentesis (0.5%).

Relative advantages of amniocentesis and CVS are outlined in Table 1. The only significant advantage of CVS is that results are available earlier in pregnancy. CVS is not as widely available as amniocentesis, and in order for this procedure to be offered the patient must present for prenatal care relatively early in pregnancy.

C. Serum Screening for Chromosome Abnormalities

Since only 20% to 30% of babies with Down syndrome are born to women over the age of 35 there has been interest in developing tests that can screen for this condition in

Table 1 Comparison of Amniocentesis Versus CVS for Genetic Testing

	Amniocentesis	CVS
Gestational age performed	15–18 weeks	10–12 weeks
Attributable loss rate	0.5%	1–2%
Availability	Widespread	More limited
Difficulty	Straightforward	Placenta sometimes inaccessible
Needle size	22 gauge	19–20 gauge (transabdominal)
Karyotype results	Definitive	2% placental mosaicism
Other information	AFP for NTD, ultrasound exam of fetus	Limited ultrasound information

younger women, who would traditionally not be offered diagnostic testing. Beginning in the 1980s it was recognized that several substances in a patient's blood are altered if she is carrying a fetus with Down syndrome. It has been determined that elevated maternal serum levels of HCG and inhibin-A and decreased serum levels of alpha fetoprotein and estriol are predictive of trisomy 21. Using these four analytes, as well as a woman's age, a patient-specific risk of Down syndrome can be calculated. If the risk is greater than that of a 35-year-old woman, the screen is considered positive and genetic counseling and amniocentesis are offered.

Soon after the introduction of serum screening in low-risk patients, investigators began to consider whether the test could be applied to older women as well. This approach initially was controversial, since it is customary to apply a diagnostic test (e.g., amniocentesis) to individuals who are at high risk for a disease (women over the age of 35) rather than subjecting them to a secondary screening test. However, the four serum marker tests have been shown to have a high sensitivity for trisomy 21 in this population (85% to 95%) (10). About 75% of women in the older age group have a "normal" test, meaning their risk becomes lower than that of a 35-year-old woman. The serum screen can be offered to patients who would very much like to avoid amniocentesis or CVS because of concerns about the risks, and who are willing to accept a less than 100% detection rate. Since the serum screen incorporates a woman's age in the risk calculation, the higher her age the higher the sensitivity for Down syndrome. Conversely, there is a lower chance that older women will have a normal result.

If a woman over the age of 35 chooses to undergo serum screening rather than proceeding directly to amniocentesis or CVS, it is important that detailed informed consent be obtained. It should be documented that a woman was informed that only an invasive diagnostic test such as amniocentesis or CVS can definitively show whether a fetus has normal karyotype. It should also be emphasized that serum screening tests for only two abnormal karyotypes, trisomy 21 and trisomy 18, while amniocentesis and CVS test for all abnormal karyotypes.

D. The "Genetic Sonogram"

As noted above, many women who are considered high risk for Down syndrome are reluctant to undergo an invasive diagnostic test. In recent years, it has been recognized that many fetuses with trisomy 21 have anatomical changes ("markers") that can be recognized with a detailed ultrasound exam. The most widely accepted of these markers include nuchal thickening, short nasal bone, echogenic bowel, shortened humerus or femur, echogenic intracardiac focus, and hydronephrosis. While results vary somewhat from study to study, virtually all studies have shown that if no markers are present, the chance that the fetus has Down syndrome is significantly reduced, usually by at least 50% (11). This provides enough reassurance for some couples that they decline amniocentesis. Since the sensitivity of the genetic sonogram will always be less than 100% this procedure does not replace amniocentesis as a definitive diagnostic test. An important limitation of the genetic sonogram is its dependence upon the quality of the ultrasound exam, which may vary according to the experience of the sonographer, maternal body habitus, and fetal position. As with the triple test, detailed documented counseling regarding the limitations of the genetic sonogram is important when this test is utilized.

E. First Trimester Noninvasive Screening

Since traditional serum screening is done after 15 weeks gestation, and the ultrasound markers mentioned above are applicable in the 16- to 20-week range, the noninvasive screening described so far is limited to the second trimester. Because of the drawbacks of mid-second trimester genetic diagnosis, as described earlier, there has been increasing recent interest in discovering ultrasound findings and serum markers which can be used in the first trimester. Two serum markers have shown to be associated with trisomy 21 in the fetus; an elevated maternal free β-HCG and decreased pregnancy-associated plasma protein A. Large studies involving ultrasound screening of patients in the late first trimester have shown that many fetuses with abnormal karyotypes have a thickened "nuchal translucency" (12). When serum markers are combined with rigorously standardized ultrasound measurements of the nuchal translucency, studies have shown a detection rate for trisomy 21 as high as 90%, with a false positive rate of 5% (13). Other first trimester markers that have been found to be associated with chromosome abnormalities include absent nasal bone and tricuspid regurgitation. The American College of Obstetrics and Gynecology has acknowledged the advantages of first trimester screening and considers combined first trimester screening using maternal serum and nuchal translucency measurement as an acceptable alternative to second trimester serum marker screening (14).

IV. MEDICAL RISKS OF PREGNANCY

There have been numerous studies and reviews concerning the risks of pregnancy in the mature gravida. The summary at the end of this chapter lists some of the major complications that have been documented in these studies. As many more recent reviews have pointed out, even though these risks and complications are real, their applicability to any given woman depends on many factors besides her age. Mansfield outlined in detail potential biases which tend to overstate the true medical risks of pregnancy in older women (15). These include the failure to control for medical complications which are themselves associated with age (16,17,18), the failure to recognize the fact that some adverse outcomes may be iatrogenic in this age group, and the failure to account for the changing demographics of older gravidas. As noted earlier in this article, pregnancies in older women are much more likely nowadays to be first pregnancies in "postponers" than last pregnancies in multiparous women. Current late-timed first births are more common among women who are highly educated, who postpone childbearing because of education or rewarding careers. These women are more likely to seek early prenatal care, have healthy lifestyles, and have a lower incidence of chronic diseases than older women having children in previous times who were more likely to be poor and uneducated. This better general health and earlier prenatal care has changed the complication rates in older women having children.

A. Maternal Death

Most studies have shown an increased maternal death rate in older gravidas. In studies performed in the late 1970s and early 1980s the death rate for women over 35 was about four times that in the general pregnant population (19) and for women 40 and older was sevenfold higher (20). Women in the older age group were much more likely to have major risk factors which contributed to mortality in pregnancy, i.e., hypertension, vascular disease, diabetes, and obesity. These risk factors predispose to potentially lethal complications such as pre-eclampsia, pulmonary embolus, abruption, and need for emergency cesarean—which in turn can cause hemorrhage and infection. Not only are these complications more common in older women, but their resultant mortality rate appears to be higher than in a younger woman with a similar disease. However older women contemplating a pregnancy should be encouraged by more recent studies which show no increase in maternal mortality if there are no underlying medical problems (19).

As previously noted, sociodemographic features may have contributed to many of the deaths in older women reported in older studies. For example, Rochat showed that women of non-caucasian race, who were more often afflicted by poverty, lack of education, and lack of access to health care, had four times the mortality rate of caucasian women (21). Buehler noted a 50% decrease in maternal mortality for women older than 35 in the late 70s and early 80s (22). He attributed this decrease to improved medical care and changing sociodemographics of the mothers in this age group.

B. Fetal Death

Virtually all studies show an increased fetal death rate in older women. A review by O'Reilly cites 10 studies demonstrating a sharp rise in fetal deaths after age 40 (20). Causes of death included congenital anomalies, placental insufficiency resulting in growth restriction and fetal asphyxia, preterm rupture of membranes, placenta previa, and chorioamnionitis. Some of these were explained by an age-related increase in chromosome abnormalities, hypertensive vascular disease, effects of multiparity, and low socioeconomic status, but the increase in deaths seemed to persist when controlling for these factors. A recent Canadian study showed that although the fetal death rate in older women decreased by 70% over the last 30 years, the chance of fetal death was significantly higher in older women, even after controlling for diabetes, hypertension, and abruption (23). The odds ratio for fetal death was 1.9 in women age 35 to 39 (compared to women less than 30 years old) and was 2.4 for women who were 40 or older. Fortunately, even though this study showed that the risk of fetal death was increased, the absolute number of deaths was low (six per 1000 deliveries instead of three per 1000).

C. Hypertension

Actuarial data show that outside of pregnancy, the incidence of hypertension rises with age, from 3% in women in the 20- to 34-year-old group to 13% in those aged 35 to 44. It comes as no surprise, therefore, that there is a higher incidence of pregnancy complications related to hypertension in older women. Hypertension complicates 7% of pregnancies in the general obstetric population, 10 to 20% of pregnancies of women over the age of 35, and 30% of pregnancies in women over age 40 (19,24). Older pregnant women with pre-existing hypertension are at high risk for the development of pre-eclampsia.

Other potentially serious pregnancy complications specifically related to hypertension, other than pre-eclampsia, include placental abruption and uteroplacental insufficiency. A study by Grimes demonstrated that increasing maternal age compounded the effects of hypertension on perinatal mortality (17). In that study, the perinatal mortality in older black women was 1.7 times the rate in younger women. When older women with hypertension were compared to younger women with hypertension, the relative risk for perinatal mortality in the offspring of the older women increased to 2.4. When women without hypertension were compared, the age effect disappeared. Of perinatal deaths 22 per 1000 were associated with hypertension in the younger women while 93 per 1000 were associated with hypertension in the older group.

D. Diabetes and Obesity

Gestational diabetes is two to three times as common in pregnancies of older women (19,25). Of the three most important risk factors for developing gestational diabetes (increased age, obesity, and family history) two are found more frequently in women in their late thirties and forties. Pregestational diabetes is also found more frequently in older gravidas. If uncontrolled in the first trimester, it is associated with an increased risk of miscarriage and fetal anomalies. When pregestational diabetes has been present for many years, vasculopathy may be present. This can result in uteroplacental insufficiency which in turn leads to fetal growth restriction, fetal distress, or even fetal death. If there is diabetic nephropathy preceding pregnancy, there is a greatly increased risk of pre-eclampsia with its attendant dangers to the mother and fetus. Hyperglycemia in the mother results in hyperinsulinemia in the fetus, which in turn often leads to fetal macrosomia. Thus, cesarean section or difficult vaginal delivery leading to birth injury is more common in pregnancies of diabetic women.

Even in the absence of diabetes, maternal obesity is a risk factor for fetal macrosomia with the attendant risks of birth injury to the baby and increased need for cesarean section. Obese women stand a substantially increased chance of operative complications should cesarean delivery be needed. One of the reasons that hypertension is more common in pregnancies of older women is the increased average weight of these patients. If an older woman is not overweight, her chance of having complications related to hypertension or diabetes is significantly reduced.

E. Other Medical Conditions

Advancing age is associated with in an increased incidence of a wide variety of other serious acute medical conditions, which can either complicate the course of pregnancy or have their effects exacerbated by pregnancy. For example, vascular diseases such as myocardial infarction, stroke, and thromboembolism all become more common with increasing age. Pregnancy itself can predispose to these acute events because pregnancy is a thrombogenic state, and because there is an increased work load on the heart during pregnancy. Fortunately, these events are rare even in older gravidas.

Most chronic diseases, such as those involving the kidneys, lungs, thyroid gland, and nervous system are more common in older individuals, and they can significantly impact pregnancy. The incidence of cancer and autoimmune diseases also increases with age. A careful assessment for any concurrent diseases is very important before a woman in her older childbearing ages conceives. While pregnancy is usually successful in the presence of most chronic diseases, there are some medical conditions which contraindicate pregnancy. Even if a woman is given a "clean bill of health" in a pre-pregnancy evaluation, the fact remains that a woman who is pregnant in her late thirties or forties is more prone to develop one of the rare acute but potentially serious medical problems during her pregnancy.

F. Placenta Previa and Abruption

Placenta previa has been linked in many studies with increased maternal age, increased parity, and prior cesarean section (26). As mentioned at the beginning of this chapter, older women having children in the past were typically multiparous, and often grand multiparous, thus in univariate analysis both age and parity were found to be risk factors for placenta previa. A woman of increased age having only her first or second child has a lower risk for placenta previa, but recent studies suggest that age persists as a risk factor, even in women of low parity (27).

Several studies have demonstrated an increased incidence of placental abruption in women over the age of 40 (20). Theoretically, abnormalities of the uterine vessels resulting from aging could cause premature separation of the placenta. As with many of the other pregnancy complications associated with maternal age, it is difficult to separate the effect of age from other factors for which there is a more clear association with placental abruption, that is, hypertension, multiparity, and substance abuse associated with low socioeconomic status. When controlling for these other risk factors, newer studies do not support any clear association between age and placental abruption (25)

G. Prematurity

There are data to suggest that increased maternal age is associated with an increased risk of preterm delivery. Much of the increase results from other complications which are more frequent in older mothers. These include complications of multiparity (e.g., placenta previa), hypertension (e.g., pre-eclampsia, abruption, or growth restriction) and diabetes (e.g., non-reassuring fetal status). Several studies have shown that older mothers more commonly experience premature rupture of membranes, a common cause of preterm birth. Most of these studies, however, were from the era when there was not adequate attention to other medical and sociodemographic factors which have been more directly linked to premature rupture of the membranes. There is no firm link established between increased maternal age and idiopathic preterm labor.

H. Fetal Growth Disorders

Fetal growth is dependent upon multiple factors: the genetic growth potential of the fetus, adequacy of utero-placental function, and nutritional factors in the pregnant woman. Numerous studies have shown that offspring of older women have an increased chance of having either inadequate or excessive growth. Most recent reviews have concluded that growth restriction in the fetuses of these women is more likely a consequence of other factors such as hypertension, smoking, and maternal social status (18,20,25). However, two studies showed that increased maternal age may exacerbate the effects of other risk factors for poor fetal growth (28,29). Two studies demonstrated a significant increase in macrosomic infants in older mothers, but this age effect on neonatal size disappeared after other well-established risk factors for excessive fetal growth, namely obesity, diabetes, and multiparity were controlled for (17,18).

I. Cesarean Section

Virtually every recent study of pregnancy outcomes in older women has shown an increased cesarean section rate in these women. A recent study by Ecker (30) evaluated all nulliparous women delivering at one Boston hospital in one year, and compared outcomes for women over age 40 with those who were less than 25 years old. They found that in the older age group there was a higher rate of both medically indicated and elective inductions. The cesarean rate for the older group was 43% compared to 12% for the younger women. The older women had a higher cesarean rate without labor, often because of a prior myomectomy or fetal malpresentation. A higher rate of fetal distress and dystocia in both spontaneous and induced labors also contributed to the increased number of cesareans in the older women.

While there is no single overriding reason that older women have more cesarean deliveries a number of factors contribute. First, as previously discussed there is an increased risk of medical and pregnancy complications which can lead to the need for cesarean section. Older women are more likely to have primary medical conditions which can cause fetal compromise or abnormal growth, pregnancy complications which may contraindicate labor, or a previous scarred uterus from a prior cesarean or myomectomy. Secondly, as discussed by Mansfield (15), some of the risk may be iatrogenic. The physician and/or older patient may be more likely to view this as a "premium pregnancy" and be more anxious about the fetal status. They may be less willing to allow the normal processes of labor to proceed and may have a lower threshold for intervening. A third component of the increased cesarean rate is that the physiology of the uterus may be altered as women age. Studies have suggested an increased incidence of dysfunctional labor patterns in older women (25), and a higher incidence of dystocia has been observed, both in spontaneous and induced labors. Non-pregnant women have been shown to have an increase in sclerotic lesions of the intramyometrial arteries as they reach their late 30s (29). If these lesions are present also in pregnancy, they could result in an increased need for cesarean delivery because of placental insufficiency.

J. Multiple Gestation

Increased maternal age has been shown to be associated with a modest increase in the spontaneous conception of multiple fetuses. With the increase in assisted reproductive technologies (ART), there has been an explosive increase in the number of twins and higher order multiples occurring in older couples. For example, for women aged 40 to 44 the twin pregnancy rate increased by 63% in 1995 compared to 1980. The rate of triplet pregnancies of women in this age group increased over 10-fold (31).

Multiple gestation increases the rate of many of the complications discussed in the preceding sections. The cardiovascular system of an older woman would be further stressed by the increased blood volume and cardiac work load imposed by multiple gestation. Pregnancy-related alterations in the hormonal milieu, which are responsible for pre-eclampsia and gestational diabetes, are even more exaggerated in multiple gestation. Increased maternal age and multiple gestation would be expected to synergistically increase the risk of these problems. Growth disorders are more common in multiple gestations, and age may, as we have shown, compound any other risk factor for poor fetal growth. Older women who conceive multiples should be made fully aware of the potentially devastating consequences of prematurity, which constitutes the most important complication of multiple gestation.

V. RECOMMENDATIONS FOR PREGNANCY MANAGEMENT

A. Preconception Preparation

Preparation for pregnancy is important for any woman, and is critical for a woman with medical risk factors. Older women contemplating a pregnancy should have a prepregnancy consultation with a physician so that risks can be identified, discussed, and modified, if possible. Some risk factors for an adverse outcome, such as age itself, multiparity, or a poor obstetrics history, cannot be modified. Obesity, which impacts on the risk of hypertension and diabetes during pregnancy can be reduced or eliminated prior to pregnancy. Cigarette smoking should be stopped prior to conception, and poor nutritional habits should be corrected. Women of all ages should take prenatal vitamins including at least 400 micrograms of folate per day, as this has been shown to reduce the incidence of neural tube defects.

Chronic medical diseases should be brought under good control, since this will minimize their impact on pregnancy. A woman should review with her physician all of her medications so that those with teratogenic potential can be eliminated. A woman's immunity to preventable viral infections should be assessed at the time of the preconception visit, and immunizations should be offered if a woman is susceptible to rubella or varicella. Hepatitis B immunization is also available for those with risk factors for blood-borne disease. The HIV status should be assessed in at-risk patients.

A woman should be informed about the genetic and medical risks which can be anticipated in a proposed pregnancy. She should be given the figures specific for her age regarding the risk of a chromosome abnormality, and options for genetic testing should be discussed. Some couples may be interested in exploring available options for reducing the risk of a chromosome abnormality in the fetus; i.e., in vitro fertilization with the pre-implantation genetic evaluation of embryos or in vitro fertilization with donor oocytes. Patients contemplating assisted reproductive technologies should be informed of the risks which would arise if they conceive multiple fetuses. Risks that are uncovered during the pre-pregnancy evaluation, as well as an overview of the counseling that was given should be documented in the patient's chart.

B. Pregnancy Care

At the first prenatal visit, the couple should be asked about their preferences for genetic testing, and appropriate appointments for counseling and procedures should be made. Because of the higher incidence of anembryonic gestations with older women, it is appropriate to perform transvaginal ultrasound to document fetal viability at the first prenatal visit.

Prenatal care is modified according to risk factors that are present. For example, if a woman has chronic hypertension, blood pressure monitoring, observation for signs of superimposed pre-eclampsia, and monitoring of fetal growth and well-being would be more intensive than usual. Because of the previously described increase in the incidence of gestational diabetes in older women it seems prudent to perform a glucose challenge test in early pregnancy as well as at the traditional time in the late second trimester.

Since increasing age is associated with a small but real increase in the incidence of utero-placental insufficiency, even in the absence of other apparent risk factors, non-stress testing beginning at 36 weeks is appropriate. In the absence of signs of fetal or maternal compromise, there is no evidence that increased age is an indication for induction or elective cesarean. Women should be informed in advance, however, that medical indications for cesarean seem to be more commonly present in older women. During the pregnancy, there should be a discussion about a woman's future reproductive plans, since many women will want a sterilization procedure performed in conjunction with a cesarean or in the immediate postpartum period.

VI. SUMMARY

There is a well-quantified increased risk of chromosome abnormalities in the offspring of women as they get older. Definitive tests for the presence of a chromosome abnormality include amniocentesis (performed at 15 weeks), and CVS (performed at 10 to 12 weeks). Because these tests are invasive and carry the risk of pregnancy loss, many women may be interested in noninvasive screening using second trimester serum screening, the second trimester "genetic sonogram," or first trimester combined nuchal translucency/serum marker screening. If normal, these noninvasive tests reduce the chance that the child is affected.

There is a long list of medical complications which has been associated with increased maternal age. These are summarized on Table 2, along with other medical

Table 2 Pregnancy Complications Associated with Increased Maternal Age. Conditions Listed in Parentheses are Predisposing Factors Which are Themselves Associated with Increased Age

- **Maternal death** (hypertensive diseases, stroke, thromboembolus, abruption, placenta previa, cesarean section, concurrent medical conditions).
- **Fetal distress or fetal death** (hypertensive diseases, vascular disease, abruption, diabetes, multiple gestation from ART).
- **Hypertensive diseases** (pre-existing hypertension, obesity).
- **Diabetes** (pre-existing diabetes, obesity).
- **Fetal macrosomia** (maternal obesity, diabetes).
- **Placenta previa** (multiparity, prior cesarean).
- **Abruption** (hypertension, vascular disease, fibroids).
- **Premature delivery** (Multiple gestation due to ART, hypertensive diseases, abruption, uteroplacental insufficiency, placenta previa, fibroids).
- **Fetal growth disorders** (hypertension, vascular disease, multiple gestation from ART).
- **Increased cesarean rate** (macrosomia from diabetes, maternal obesity, placenta previa, abruption, fetal distress from hypertensive diseases or vascular disease, multiple gestation from ART).
- **Increased rate of hospitalization** (chronic hypertension leading to pre-eclampsia and abruption, diabetes with admission for glucose control, placenta previa, multiple gestation with preterm labor, degenerating fibroids).

conditions which are themselves associated with increased maternal age and which predispose a woman to the listed complication.

An older women planning a pregnancy should have a pre-pregnancy evaluation so that risk factors can be identified, and modified, if possible. She should be fully appraised of the genetic and medical risks. Most women in the older age groups can have a successful pregnancy, especially if there are no pre-existing medical conditions which contribute to the risks. Management of pregnancy is individualized according to specific risks that are identified. In most instances, however, it will be appropriate to offer genetic testing of the fetus, perform more intensive screening for gestational diabetes, and perform tests of fetal well-being near term.

REFERENCES

1. Births: Final Data for 1999. National Vital Statistics Report, 1999; 49(1).
2. Ventura SJ. Trends in first births to older mothers. National Center for Health Statistics 1970–79. 1982; 31(2) Supplement (2).
3. Live births by age of mother, live-birth order, and race of mother: United States, 2000. National Vital Statistics Report 2002; 50(5).
4. Backu A, O'Connell M. Fertility of American women: June 2000. U.S. Census Bureau, Current Population Reports, issued October 2001.
5. Hook EB. Rates of chromosome abnormalities at different maternal ages. Obstet Gynecol 1981; 58:282–285.
6. The Canadian Early and Mid-trimester Amniocentesis Trial (CEMAT) Group. Randomised trial to assess safety and fetal outcome of early and mid trimester amniocentesis. Lancet 1998; 351:242–247.
7. Blessed WB, Lacoste H, Welch RA. Obstetrician-gynecologists performing genetic amniocentesis may be misleading themselves and their patients. Am J Obstet Gynecol 2001; 184:1342–1344.

8. Wilson RD. Amniocentesis and chorionic villus sampling. Curr Opin Obstet Gynecol 2000; 12:81–86.

9. Scott F, Peters H, Boogert T et al. The loss rates for invasive prenatal testing in a specialized obstetric ultrasound practice. Aust N Z J Obstet Gynaecol 2002 Feb; 42:55–58.

10. Haddow JE, Palomaki GE, Knight GJ et al. Reducing the need for amniocentesis in women 35 years of age or older with serum markers for screening. N Engl J Med 1994; 330: 1114–1118.

11. Nyberg DA, Luthy DA, Resta RG et al. Age-adjusted ultrasound risk assessment for fetal Down's syndrome during the second trimester: Description of the method and analysis of 142 cases. Ultrasound Obstet Gynecol 1998; 12:8–14.

12. Taipale P, Hiilesma V, Salonen R et al. Increased nuchal translucency as a marker of fetal chromosomal defects. N Engl J Med 1997; 337:1654–1658.

13. Nicolaides, KH. Nuchal translucency and other first-trimester sonographic markers of chromosomal abnormalities. Am J Obstet Gynecol 2004; 191:47–65.

14. First-trimester screening for fetal aneuploidy. ACOG Committee Opinion Number 296, 2004.

15. Mansfield PK, McCool W. Toward a better understanding of the "advanced maternal age" factor. Health Care for Women Intl 1989; 10:395–415.

16. Dildy GA, Jackson GM, Fowers GK. Very advanced maternal age: Pregnancy after age 45. Am J Obstet Gynecol 1996; 175:668–674.

17. Grimes DA, Gross GK. Pregnancy outcomes in black women aged 35 and older. Obstet Gynecol 1981; 58:614–620.

18. Spellacy WN, Miller J, Winegar A. Pregnancy after 40 years of age. Obstet Gynecol 1986; 68:452–454.

19. Cunningham FG, Leveno KJ. Childbearing among older women—the message is cautiously optimistic. N Engl J Med 1995; 333:1002–1004.

20. O'Reilly-Green C, Cohen WR. Pregnancy in women aged 40 and older. Perimenopausal Health Care 1993; 20:313–331.

21. Rochat RW, Koonin LM, Atrash HK et al. Maternal mortality in the United States: Report from the Maternal Mortality Collaborative. Obstet Gynecol 1988; 72:91–97.

22. Buehler JW, Kaunitz AM, Hogue CJR et al. Maternal mortality in women aged 35 years or older: United States. JAMA 1986; 255:53–57.

23. Fretts RC, Schmittdiel J, McLean FH et al. Increased maternal age and the risk of fetal death. N Engl J Med 1995; 333(15):1002–1004.

24. Kajanoja P, Widholm O. Pregnancy and delivery in women aged 40 and over. Obstet Gynecol 1978; 51:47–51.

25. Fonteyn VJ, Isada NB. Nongenetic implications of childbearing after age 35. Obstet Gynecol Surv 1988; 43:709–719.

26. Clark SL, Koonings PP, Phelan JP. Placenta previa/accreta and prior cesarean section. Obstet Gynecol 1985; 66:89–92.

27. Rasmussen S, Albrechtsen S, Dalaker K. Obstetric history and the risk of placenta previa. Acta Obstet Gynecol Scand 2000; 79:402–507.

28. Cnattingius S, Forman ME, Berendes HW et al. Delayed childbearing and risk of adverse perinatal outcome. A population-based study. JAMA 1992; 268:886–890.

29. Naeye RL. Maternal age, obstetric complications, and the outcome of pregnancy. Obstet Gynecol 1983; 61:210–216.

30. Ecker JL, Chen KT, Cohen AP et al. Increased risk of cesarean delivery with advancing maternal age: Indications and associated factors in nulliparous women. Am J Obstet Gynecol 2001; 185:883–887.

31. Martin JA, Park MM. Trends in twin and triplet births. National Vital Statistics Report 1999; 47(24).

6

Psychological Disorders in the Perimenopause

Shae Graham Kosch
Behavioral Medicine Program, Department of Community Health and Family Medicine, University of Florida College of Medicine, Gainesville, Florida, U.S.A.

Karen L. Hall
Department of Community Health and Family Medicine, University of Florida College of Medicine, Gainesville, Florida, U.S.A.

I. INTRODUCTION

A. Evidence-based Approach to Perimenopausal Symptoms and Treatment

The North American Menopause Society (NAMS), in developing a consensus opinion in 2000 for clinical management of perimenopausal problems, stated that there was inadequate clinical trial data to formulate evidence-based treatment protocols for women in this life phase (1). At that point in time, then, clinicians were left with using data on menopausal women and translating those findings back to women in the perimenopause or relying on their clinical experience in developing treatment approaches for patients. Subsequent to that, NAMS updated position statements over the years and established more precise, evidence-based guidelines in 2007 for women in the perimenopausal phase (2). Many changes or problems reported by perimenopausal women are similar to those of diagnosed emotional disorders with depressive or anxiety symptoms—insomnia, fatigue, low mood, tension, concentration and memory problems. It is important for clinicians to distinguish between expected changes in the climacteric phase and symptoms that meet criteria for emotional disorders.

For healthy middle-aged women without prior psychiatric problems, the time frame from perimenopause to menopause appears to be a benign transition (3,4). Although many women experience physical and psychological changes in natural peri/postmenopause that are similar to signs of emotional disorders, these symptoms are manageable, do not cause any long-term change in psychological function, and remit spontaneously with time (3–8). The bulk of the evidence suggests that the prevalence of true emotional disorders is not increased in the perimenopause and experienced emotional distress may be linked to other factors, such as social stressors (9). It is important to emphasize that the somatic and mental symptoms of perimenopause are distinct from psychopathology. Clinicians should not conceptualize these as closely linked together into some type of pathological symptom constellation of a climacteric transition. On the other hand, studies indicate that patients with a previous diagnosis of an emotional disorder may have an exacerbation of their underlying disorder during this time frame.

B. Incidence of Symptoms and Emotional Disorders in the Perimenopause

A multitude of studies have surveyed the somatic and psychologic complaints of women in the perimenopausal transition through the climacteric (3–8,10–23). Deriving solid conclusions from these studies is difficult due to the utilization of diverse methodological approaches. The studies were similar in that they employed primarily self-report measures of anxiety and depression, as well as scales aimed at a global assessment of well-being and perceptions of health. Several of the studies are prospective (3,4,11,14,15,19,24); represent women studied in Europe, Australia, and the United States, and include cross-cultural data (11,25). One of the major issues in summarizing the findings from these studies lies in the selection of different patient populations. Not surprisingly, studies based on populations seeking medical care or attending menopause clinics report greater symptom complexes in their patient populations than those projects that surveyed general populations of women (21,26). The clinic-based studies reported greater distress with the menopausal transition and more psychological complaints. For instance, one study of women attending a menopause clinic reported increased anxiety in perimenopausal women when compared with postmenopausal women (21). Several studies emphasized the link between prior medical or psychiatric conditions and poorer overall functioning to the severity of distress experienced in the perimenopause. Hunter and colleagues reported increased depressed mood in perimenopausal and menopausal patients in their sample; past depression and social factors correlated with the presence of symptoms in just over half of the patients (22). Morse concluded that a history of prior premenstrual complaints predicted greater distress with menopause (15). Neri and colleagues reported that perimenopausal symptoms were affected by biological, social, and "personal resource" variables (27). Other studies commented on the length of the perimenopause and noted that a greater number of symptoms occur in those patients who experience a longer transition to menopause (28). This is similar to the findings of increased depressive symptoms with a lengthy perimenopause in the Massachusetts Women's Health Study (3,29). It is important to underscore that the Study of Women's Health Across the Nation (SWAN) documented that all minority group perimenopausal women (African-American, Hispanic, Chinese, and Japanese) in a total cohort of over 16,000 women had significantly lower levels of distress than Caucasians (25).

II. PREVALENCE OF EMOTIONAL DISORDERS THROUGHOUT THE LIFECYCLE

Several survey studies provide an overview of mental disorders in the United States. The largest of these are two population-based studies, the Epidemiologic Catchment Area Survey (ECA), conducted by the National Institute of Mental Health (30,31) in the 1980s and the National Comorbidity Survey (NCS), conducted in the early 1990s (32). It is difficult to compare the findings from each of these projects to each other and to later studies, as the diagnostic categories vary across the projects, as do the study samples.

For instance, the ECA included institutionalized populations and focused on particular anxiety disorders and not others that were included in later surveys. NCS sampled patients from 15 to 54 years of age and included some of the same anxiety disorders as the ECA, but excluded others. The criteria for depression across both studies had less variability, but still included different study populations and methodology. Both of these epidemiological surveys report an increased prevalence of both depression and anxiety disorders in women compared with men throughout the lifecycle. Although the projects did not specifically investigate menstrual status, there was not a reported increase in the incidence of emotional disorders among women in the age groups usually associated with the perimenopause.

A. Criteria for Disorders and Screening Instruments to Assess Emotional Disorders

1. Major Affective Disorder, Unipolar Depression

According to Diagnostic and Statistical Manual of Mental Disorders, IV edition (DSM IV) (32a) criteria, a patient diagnosed with major affective disorder (unipolar depression) must display either anhedonia or dysphoria, as well as a total of five or more symptoms from the following list during a two-week period, and the symptoms must indicate a change from previous levels of functioning: (1) ahedonia, or loss of interest or pleasure in almost all activities; (2) dysphoria (depressed mood) most every day, often with diurnal variation involving feeling worse in the morning; (3) insomnia (often early morning wakening) or hypersomnia; (4) fatigue or loss of energy; (5) decreased concentration, indecisiveness, cognitive or memory problems; (6) significant weight loss or weight gain; (7) feelings of worthlessness or excessive guilt; (8) psychomotor agitation or retardation; and (9) recurrent thoughts of death or suicide. In terms of the differential diagnosis of major depressive disorder, the clinician must distinguish it from dysthymic disorder, adjustment disorder with depressed mood or mixed emotional features, depression associated with organic syndromes, and uncomplicated bereavement. The symptoms of dysthymic disorder are less severe than major affective disorder and include problems with appetite, insomnia, fatigue, low self-esteem, poor concentration, and feelings of hopelessness, which persist for a two-year or longer time period without a clear symptom-free period. It is also important to note that about 30% of depressed patients also experience significantly elevated anxiety and have "overlap" syndromes of both depression and anxiety (33). Both anxiety and depression often include symptoms of insomnia, changes in appetite, increased irritability, fatigue, and gastrointestinal or cardiopulmonary symptoms. Patients may present to physicians with physical symptoms, rather than emotional ones, with patterns of ill-defined somatic symptoms, pain of unknown etiology, and "nervous" complaints such as increased tension.

2. The Anxiety Disorders

In discussing criteria for the diagnosis of one of the anxiety disorders, it is important to separate the general term of "anxiety" from the concept of discrete anxiety disorders as defined in the DSM-IV. Anxiety is a sense of apprehension or uneasiness, and is, in its mild state, a nearly universal component of human consciousness. Anxiety disorders as defined by the DSM-IV are discrete mental disorders where the state of anxiety is of such a degree that it significantly compromises normal functioning. These specific disorders are currently categorized as generalized anxiety disorder (GAD), panic disorder—with and without agoraphobia, agoraphobia alone, acute stress disorder, post-traumatic stress disorder (PTSD), obsessive compulsive disorder (OCD), adjustment disorder with anxious mood and anxiety associated with organic illness or substance abuse. Incapacitating anxiety is a key component of these disorders, and interference with normal functioning is required for diagnosis (see the DSM-IV for criteria). A brief description of each disorder may under-score the severity and chronicity of the symptoms of anxiety disorders and distinguish them from the normal experience of anxiety. In GAD, the central symptoms involve excessive or unrealistic worry about events on a daily basis, an inability to cease or control the worry, and the presence of at least three other symptoms of sleep disorder, muscle tension or restlessness, irritability, fatigue, or a type of cognitive process that focuses on catastrophe events or the possibility of injury to oneself or one's loved ones. Although the person may be "on edge" or nervous and may have "anxiety attacks," the cognitive symptoms predom-inate. Panic disorder, on the other hand, has a dominance of somatic symptoms. During "panic attacks," in which the person may experience dyspnea, tachycardia, numbness or tingling, dizziness, or diaphoresis, the symptoms may be attributed to a serious physical illness, such as a heart attack or other lethal event. In terms of cognitive components, the person may be afraid that they will do something extreme during the event, such as yell uncontrollably or lose muscle control in a public place. The anticipation of the next attack is a hallmark sign of panic disorder, and a person may become so fearful of these occur-ring that they feel afraid of being out in public and become home-bound (agoraphobia). PTSD refers to an acute or chronic reaction, with dominant symptoms of anxiety, that occurs subsequent to a frightening event, such as a fire or a rape, or a series of events (chronic child abuse). PTSD has symptoms of flashbacks, nightmares, depersonalization, and a heightened vigilance about danger associated with it. OCD is a condition character-ized by excessive anxiety, marked by repetitive, intrusive thoughts that the person tries to manage by ritualistic behavior or a high level of organization. Adjustment disorder with anxious mood is a condition in which a person has a period of elevated anxiety due to a change in life situation (a change in employment, geographic relocation, a personal loss) that is time-limited and less severe than the symptoms of GAD. It is also important to dis-tinguish anxiety from irritability or tension. Although irritability is a frequent symptom of generalized anxiety disorder, it may exist as a separate phenomenon from an anxiety dis-order. Patients who are irritable may be easily annoyed or provoked and lacking in patience, but they are not necessarily anxious. Some symptoms of the perimenopause such as insomnia or sleep disturbance may cause or worsen both irritability and anxiety.

3. Psychometric Scales in the Diagnosis of Anxiety or Depression

For research purposes, the assessment of depression or anxiety is often completed by clinicians or researchers interviewing patients extensively about their symptom complexes, using such scales as a Hamilton Depression Scale or a Center for Epidemiologic Studies scale for Depression (CES-D). Patients may also be asked to complete paper and pencil instruments to collect information about their perception of symptoms. Busy clinicians can use self-report screening scales to assess the possibility of depression or anxiety in patients—these have been shown to be highly sensitive and reliable instruments and can be used to determine the potential benefit of treatment by repeat administration after instituting a therapeutic regimen. Scales in this category include the Beck Depression Inventory-II (34), the Zung Self-Rating Depression Scale (35), and the Zung Self-Rating Anxiety Scale (36). For the detection of depression, both the Beck and Zung scales have been shown to be very effective, with a high level of sensitivity and specificity (37) and correlated with other scales that clinicians may find even easier to use in primary care practice (38). Several pharmaceutical companies provide physicians with these scales in an easy format for patient assessment and scoring.

B. Prevalence and Diagnosis of Depression Throughout the Life Span

The lifetime prevalence of diagnosed mood disorders over all years was estimated to be approximately 17% in the ECA study. Symptoms of dysphoria are a common presentation of women during the climacteric period of life, but there is no evidence of an increased incidence in major affective disorder according to criteria established by the DSM-IV. It is unclear whether many women experience subsyndromal depression or adjustment disorder with depressed mood during perimenopause. Other reports estimated that depression involves 10 million people yearly in the United States, based on National Institute of Mental Health figures and that a lifetime incidence of major depression may be as high as 50% (39,40). In primary care practices, depression has been shown to have a 6% to 8% point prevalence (41). The possibility of an increase in depression as result of hormonal changes has been well-studied, but the results are contradictory. Burt, et al. note the paucity of studies that document the incidence of major depressive disorder in perimenopausal women (42), but did report an association between depressive symptoms and the perimenopause, especially for women with a past history of the disorder. Schmidt et al., concluding that the literature is inconclusive, cited a variety of epidemiologic studies showing that the majority of women did not develop depression during the perimenopause and other epidemiologic or clinic-based studies reporting that a substantial number of perimenopausal women did have unipolar depression (43). In order to resolve the contradictory conclusions in the literature, the authors suggest that it would be important to design studies that can isolate factors that may influence the development of mood disorders during the mid-life period.

In one community-based project, the self-reporting of depressed mood was shown to be 36% for women in the premenopause, 47% for perimenopause, and 46% for postmenopause; whereas it was 37%, 47%, and 60% respectively, for insomnia and 58%, 68%, and 68%, for tiredness (12). These findings would suggest that depression was higher in this perimenopausal sample than a point prevalence in the general population would predict; however, the samples did not include a much younger cohort as a comparison sample, so a definitive comparison cannot be achieved. Another prospective population-based study (14) found the rate of self-reported depression at 26%, 26%, and 38% for the same three phases of the climacteric, and sleeping problems were recorded at 31%, 32%, and 38%. Fatigue was a greater problem than either depression or sleep disruption in this study, experienced by 42% of perimenopausal and 43% of premenopausal and postmenopausal women. Other reports of general population samples have found no increase in depression, poor psychological status, or sleep disturbance associated with the perimenopause or menopause compared to premenopausal women (44). Other researchers have investigated the role of disturbed sleep in the genesis of psychological symptoms seen in the perimenopausal time frame (45–47). In the SWAN study, psychologic distress correlated highly with the presence of sleep disturbance and vasomotor symptoms. In addition, psychologic distress was higher in patients in the perimenopause transition than in premenopausal or postmenopausal patients regardless of the presence of sleep or vasomotor symptoms. This would indicate that other factors in addition to sleep and vasomotor symptoms are responsible for the distress in the perimenopausal patient (25). Li et al., using quality of life and health assessment scales, found that a greater number of perimenopausal women reported psychosomatic complaints than vasomotor symptoms (48). However, they also identified an important mediating factor—activity level. In inquiring about the women's physical activity level, they determined that women who were moderately to very active had fewer psychological symptoms of distress, such as irritability, memory problems, headaches, and sexual symptoms, whereas activity level was not related to problems with vasomotor or menstrual symptoms.

C. Prevalence and Diagnosis of Anxiety Disorders Throughout the Lifecycle

In terms of anxiety disorders, there is no firm evidence that aging or the middle years increase the incidence of these disorders in women. Anxiety disorders generally tend to be lifelong, with dominant symptoms appearing in a woman's 20s and 30s and persisting into the peri- and postmenopausal periods as well as the geriatric period. It is also noteworthy that recent research has indicated that many children have clear symptoms of social phobia or generalized anxiety disorder, confirming the idea that even younger people may have a definite constellation of symptoms that simply may not be diagnosed as an anxiety disorder until they are adults. As anxiety disorders are more common in women than men throughout the lifecycle (49–51), it would seem plausible that anxiety disorders could be exacerbated by changes in endocrine balance during the perimenopause. However, the Epidemiologic Catchment Area Survey (ECA) and the National Comorbidity Survey (NCS) did not report an increase of anxiety disorders in typical perimenopausal age groups, rather both report a decline in prevalence of anxiety disorders with advancing age (52). The NCS reports the highest prevalence of anxiety disorders in the 15- to 24-year-old age group (10). In the ECA study, one-month prevalence of anxiety disorders drops in the 45- to 64-year-age group (52). Overall, the ECA survey noted a lifetime prevalence of anxiety disorders for U.S. adults of 14.6%; furthermore, at any one time, it was estimated that approximately 12.5 million people suffer from a treatable anxiety disorder. One report noted a 25% lifetime prevalence of an anxiety disorder in the general population and underscored that these disorders cause significant morbidity and an annual mortality of 3% (53). The rate of untreated anxiety disorders is also significant, with estimates that fewer than 25% ever receive appropriate treatment.

Several reports based on ECA and NCS data note the onset of anxiety disorders in younger age cohorts as opposed to middle-aged persons (40,54,55). In a community-based sample, Maartens and colleagues reported no significant elevation of anxiety in their perimenopausal group; although irritability and agitation were common, they were not significantly different from pre- to peri- to postmenopausal patient groups (12). Several population-based studies did report higher levels of anxiety in perimenopausal patients (11,14,17). Two reports found that anxiety was higher in pre- or perimenopausal patients but was linked to depression rather than standing alone (13,24). Other authors note that it is common for symptoms of anxiety to be transient in the perimenopausal period and to resolve by the menopause (6,21). In general, then, data do not support the concept of an increase in the prevalence of discrete anxiety disorders in perimenopausal women, as these are conditions that evolve earlier and persist over the lifecycle, but women may experience transitory increased symptoms of anxiety during this life phase.

D. Cognitive Functioning in the Perimenopause

Recent work has focused on the possible connection between neurodegeneration and "brain aging" and ovarian failure. Changes in memory, ischemic brain events, and Alzheimer's disease are all possible sequelae of estrogen deficiency. Some evidence exists that estrogen can affect cognition and memory functions by an influence on brain architecture, as well as on multiple neurotransmitters (56). Although there is contradictory data in the research literature, it appears that estrogen has a beneficial effect on some aspects of memory (57). Lichtman's literature review, however, concludes that there is no evidence that perimenopausal women have any memory loss that impairs their ability to function (58). Although evidence from controlled studies is inconclusive, some studies have shown that estrogen replacement may prevent women from developing Alzheimer's disease and/or improve the functioning of those with the disease (59,60). Other observational studies have suggested a later development in Alzheimer's disease in women on HRT; but no effect on the disease once it is present (61). Data from the Women's Health Initiative indicated that older women taking estrogen only, as well as estrogen plus progestin, could have a slightly increased risk of cognitive problems and development of dementia than women who did not use any hormonal therapy (61a).

E. Menstrual Symptoms and Premenstrual Syndrome

Almost all women experience significant changes in menstrual patterns during the perimenopause, with a first dynamic of a shorter cycle with increased menstrual flow or cramping and a later dynamic of a longer cycle with lighter bleeding. Whether premenstrual symptoms or premenstrual syndrome (PMS) is more frequent is the subject of debate. One prospective study of perimenopausal women found a clear relationship between having significant premenstrual complaints prior to the initiation of ovarian failure and having them during the perimenopause (15). Other projects have also documented that women who have experienced psychological symptoms during the premenstrual phase of their menstrual cycles may be at increased risk of experiencing psychological problems during the perimenopause (22). Contrary to this, some reports have noted that most women do not experience significant difficulties with menstruation or changes in the perimenopause (62). The influence of psychological and social events during the midlife period may be more predictive of self-perceived symptoms in women than menstrual or hormonal changes (63,64).

F. Contribution of Sociocultural and Interpersonal Factors

Attitudes toward aging and beliefs about menopause vary from culture to culture and all women do not universally experience the symptoms often associated with the climacteric in the medical literature in the United States. For instance, one study reported that African-American women reported more vasomotor symptoms, while Caucasian women described more psychological symptoms (11). Investigators have also reported greater symptoms in Caucasian women in comparison to other cultural groups (25,65). It is also crucial to acknowledge that perimenopausal women may experience increased stressors or psychosocial changes that have the potential to impact mood. Many reports cite a correlation between psychological symptoms in the peri/postmenopausal time frames and social concerns or life stressors—such as divorce or death of a spouse; difficulty with children or children leaving home; increased demands of aging or ill parents; or facing their own aging process (7,10,15,17,22,23,27,66). These findings suggest that concomitant life stressors can be cofactors with organic and/or endocrine changes in the genesis of anxiety or depression in the perimenopause.

III. TREATMENT AND MANAGEMENT OF PSYCHOLOGICAL DISORDERS IN THE PERIMENOPAUSE

A. Behavioral and Contextual Treatment of Emotional Disorders

1. Psychoeducation and Bibliotherapy

For patients to adhere to a treatment program and to learn "self-calming" techniques or "mood-elevating" techniques, they must clearly understand both the physiological and the psychological aspects of their disorders. One of the most important aspects for the clinician to stress is that emotional disorders are not "all in the mind"; rather, the disorders exist in both mind and body. It is crucial to emphasize that they are clearly psychosomatic or somatopsychic disorders with physical, physiological, as well as cognitive and emotional components. This idea is especially important to stress for well-educated patients, who may believe that they should be able to alter an anxiety disorder or depression with "will power" or that they are "weak" if they use psychotropic medications. On the other hand, some other patients, possibly more highly represented in less educated groups, believe that they have "bad nerves" and that their symptoms are all physical and can only be treated with a "nerve pill." It is essential to inform these patients about the critical role of psychological and behavioral components in order to get them to participate in counseling and lifestyle modification. Good resources for self-help in the areas of depression (67,68), anxiety, and panic disorder (69) are available. Patient education materials also are available for obsessive-compulsive disorder (70). Patients with anxiety disorders benefit from having anxiety symptoms "normalized" as being a common part of human experience and told that coping skills can effectively deal with these symptoms. As Beck and Emery pointed out, as patients focus on anxiety symptoms, the symptoms become stronger, creating a circular spiral (71). They suggest that the clinician explain this phenomenon and give patients techniques to minimize, rather than maximize the symptoms. "Anxiety consists of those symptoms we have talked about—dizziness, light-headedness, tightness in the throat, a variety of palpitations, sweating, and so on. You often start worrying about these symptoms. You then label them as dangerous, a warning that something terrible is about to happen. This creates more anxiety. The more anxious you become, the more the symptoms increase, It becomes circular because you are focusing too much on these symptoms." (71: p. 237). These therapists state that patients benefit from the understanding that these symptoms once served a purpose in humans, when they were needed to avoid real environmental threats (such as large bears in the woods); this is referred to as the "evolutionary model of anxiety."

B. Lifestyle Variables

Any patient who requires treatment for emotional disorders must be evaluated for the contribution of lifestyle factors, including dietary patterns, substance use, exercise patterns, sleep patterns, stressors, and social support systems. For women with mild to moderate depressive symptoms or minor anxiety, good sleep hygiene, a balanced diet, and routine exercise are appropriate prescriptions. As disturbances of sleep are a frequent part of the presentation in anxiety or depressive states, as well as the perimenopause, and are profoundly affected by daily patterns, it is essential that a treatment strategy include investigation and modification of problematic areas. As an extreme example, it is folly to prescribe an agent for sleep induction to a patient who ingests 10 cups of coffee per day without first having them reduce or eliminate the caffeine intake. "Common sense" suggestions of the avoidance/moderate use of caffeine, nicotine, alcohol, or other drugs and over- or undereating are often helpful in the management of anxiety and depression. One aspect to note is the creation of panic attacks in patients with panic disorder by infusion of a lactic acid solution and their control by calcium. Calcium metabolism may be essential to the occurrence of panic symptoms, and yet a history of dietary calcium intake or caffeine intake is often not included as part of the work-up for these patients. Obviously, patients with more serious lifestyle problems should be referred to programs for smoking cessation, addiction treatment, or eating disorder counseling.

1. Exercise is Associated with Lowered Risk of Depression and Anxiety

Several studies emphasize the importance of exercise for a sense of well-being in general, and in alleviating perimenopausal symptoms in particular (72–74). Slaven and Lee reported reduction in both vasomotor and somatic symptoms following aerobic exercise as well as improved mood among women who exercised compared with sedentary women (74) There is also data to support the efficacy of aerobic exercise in the treatment of mild depression and a clear association between a sedentary lifestyle and higher symptoms of depression and anxiety in women (75). Li et al. concluded that moderate to high levels of exercise lowered symptoms of psychological distress and might be an effective alternative to pharmacotherapy for perimenopausal psychological symptoms (48). They did note no impact on vasomotor or menstrual symptoms. Extrapolating from these types of projects, it is reasonable to view exercise as a powerful treatment modality, even one that could be considered the "fountain of youth" (76,77).

2. Biopsychosocial Approach to Insomnia

Disordered sleep is a significant symptom in both anxiety disorders and depression, as well as being a dominant symptom in peri- and postmenopausal women. Morin and Kwentus clearly detail the enormity of the problem of insomnia and its treatment (78). They estimate that between 15% and 30% of the U.S. adult population complain of insomnia; many of these patients use either over-the-counter medications or prescribed hypnotics, which usually offer benefits for less than four weeks of continuous use. They cite moderate clinical benefits for treating onset insomnia with relaxation techniques and biofeedback, noting improvement rates from 40% to 60% for sleep latency. Cognitive interventions offer improvement in the 50% to 60% range. In addition to the behavioral and contextual treatments listed in the previous text, there are certain "rules" about sleep induction and maintenance that should be suggested to patients. The stimulus control procedures developed by Bootzin and Rider have been shown to have mean reductions of 65% in sleep onset latency, 60% reduction in the duration of awake periods, and 35% reduction in numbers of awakenings (79,80). The information contained in the attached chart (Table 1) can be offered to patients as a behavioral prescription for better sleep hygiene that will improve sleep onset, maintenance, and quality.

Table 1 How to Improve Your Rest by Good Sleep Hygiene

1. Get up at the same time every morning, regardless of the amount of sleep obtained on the previous night.
2. Avoid daytime napping.
3. Avoid caffeine, chocolate, nicotine, and alcohol, especially close to bedtime.
4. Exercise daily (aerobic) for 45 to 60 minutes in the late afternoon (around 4 to 7 pm).
5. Use the bed only for sleep and sex (no reading, eating, TV watching, working, or worrying) either during the day or at bedtime.
6. Eat a bedtime snack of milk and cookies, cereal, or a banana.
7. Go to bed only when sleepy.
8. Use relaxation techniques or relaxing audiotapes (or CDs) after getting in bed.
9. When unable to fall asleep or return to sleep within 15 to 20 minutes, get out of bed, go in another room, and return to bed only when sleepy. Avoid exposure to light.
10. Repeat Steps 8 and 9 as often as necessary throughout the night.

C. Psychotherapy and Counseling Approaches for Anxiety and Depression

Many primary care providers prefer to refer patients to mental health practitioners for specialized, therapeutic interventions. However, it is important for women's health providers to be aware of the criteria for specific anxiety disorders and unipolar depression, so that recognition and appropriate referral are accomplished. Additionally, many patients prefer to receive services solely from their primary care providers and these providers will thus be the ones delivering counseling services. Fortunately, many effective counseling techniques are amenable to time-limited structured, outpatient medical visits.

1. Self-regulation of Anxiety and Mood

The reduction of muscular tension and the modulation of anxiety-producing and dysphoria-eliciting thoughts are effective techniques in the psychological management of anxiety, depression, and mixed anxiety-depressive disorders. Various approaches, such as progressive relaxation, autogenic training, clinical hypnosis, self-hypnosis, and biofeedback training, have been shown to be highly effective in teaching patients to regulate motor and cognitive processes and attain a state of relaxation (69). Progressive relaxation and autogenic training are approaches that teach patients deep muscular relaxation and focus cognitive processes toward calm and positive ideation. Biofeedback uses similar techniques, but provides either visual or auditory "feedback" to the patient when the monitoring equipment detects relaxation. As behaviorally oriented psychotherapists have repeatedly noted, it is impossible to experience anxiety if every muscle in the body is relaxed. Patients should participate in one of these programs as a first-line treatment; the program can be conducted by the primary care physician or the patient can be referred to a psychotherapist. Excellent audiotapes and CDs for autogenic training developed by Emmett Miller, M.D. are available online at www.drmiller.org and can be provided to patients for use outside of the medical encounter.

In terms of treatment during the perimenopause, the addition of psychological treatment to hormone replacement therapy was more effective than HRT alone in resolving insomnia, anxiety, dysphoria, fatigue, and various other somatic symptoms (81). In terms of the treatment of psychological disorders, treatment strategies for depression and anxiety can be viewed as having more similarities than differences. For instance, the essential ingredients in a cognitive behavioral approach emphasize the alteration of the patient's cognitive functioning, which results in a change in emotional responding (71,82). In the case of depression, patients are seen as having "negative, automatic thoughts," such as "I am worthless" or "I do not have the skills to achieve what I want in life" or "I am unlovable." The crux of cognitive behavioral work with a patient has the therapist urging the patient to refocus on affirmations, such as the statements "I am a competent and worthy person and have achieved many things in my life" or "I have many friends and a spouse and am indeed lovable." The idea behind this approach is that if health care providers can succeed in getting patients to alter their internal conversations about their qualities and experiences, the affective reactions that they usually have, such as sadness or a sense of hopelessness, can be transformed to more positive and esteem-building ones. In the case of an anxiety disorder, patients often ruminate about catastrophes they anticipate may occur to themselves or to loved ones, such as automobile accidents, socially embarrassing situations, or uncontrollable physical symptoms that will be observed by others (e.g., a tremor). In this case, the health care provider focuses on teaching the patient to reduce these catastrophic thoughts and substitute positive, affirmative thoughts. The absence of the negative, automatic thoughts leads to a decline in both physical and psychological symptoms of anxiety and/or depression. For particular anxiety disorders, a patient may derive definite benefit from other specialized therapeutic approaches such as in vivo exposure for OCD or specific phobias, in which the patient learns to cope successfully during exposure of anxiety-provoking situations.

The Depression Guideline Panel found that there was a level B strength of evidence for the effectiveness of psychotherapy alone for patients with moderate depression without psychosis (41). The panel stated that randomized controlled trials of psychotherapy were predominantly focused on time-limited, structured forms of psychotherapy, including cognitive, interpersonal, behavioral, brief dynamic, and marital psychotherapy. The trials have generally shown that the formal, short-term psychotherapies perform about equal to each other in outcome, are significantly superior to wait-list comparison groups, and offer an equivalent outcome to medication. Therefore, when a clinician seeks evidence-based protocols, the effective ones appear to be those that involve a structured kind of approach to psychotherapy that enables patients to produce long-standing emotional and behavioral change. Even though several approaches to psychotherapy have equal value, it may behoove primary care physicians to become familiar with cognitive behavioral therapy, as it is a time-limited, structured approach that has been well adapted for primary care practices. Providers can familiarize themselves with many aspects of a CBT approach to therapy by reading the program developed by a RAND research project called Partners in Care and adapt homework assignments from it for their practices. It can be accessed online at www.rand.org/health/partners.care/portweb/ and findings from the project in terms of outcome can be accessed at www.rand.org/health/pic.products/.

Many studies have found strong support for the effectiveness of cognitive behavioral therapy in depression (83,84) and when compared to other therapeutic modalities, with CBT performing better or as well as other modalities in most studies (85,86). In the treatment of anxiety, CBT has also been shown to have high efficacy (87) and compares favorably to other therapeutic approaches (88). In comparing cognitive behavioral therapy to pharmacotherapy, several studies over the last few years have indicated that for long-term decreases in symptom constellation, cognitive behavioral therapy is as effective or superior to medication. As an example, cognitive behavior therapy had the highest improvement in reducing or eliminating depressive symptoms at the end of a 24-month post-treatment follow-up period; the relapse rate for medication and standard clinical management was 80%, while CBT had a 20% relapse rate (89). Another study of severely depressed outpatients with a 12-month follow-up of patients who had 16 weeks of either cognitive therapy or pharmacotherapy documented that CBT offered continued improvement greater to or equal to medication at less cost (90). With the availability of generics, the cost comparison is less relevant today.

As noted by Holmes in a critique of evidence-based medicine in general, and the reliance on CBT in the treatment of depression in particular, the choice of CBT in research protocols may be driven by the ability of CBT to fit within the randomized, placebo-controlled model used to study the efficacy of medications (91). Holmes contended that several other psychotherapeutic modalities may be equally or more effective than CBT, but are less suited to the research design that is now seen as the "gold standard" of evidence-based medicine. In other words, the research method may dictate the modality of treatment, and researchers may simply not be collecting important data about potentially efficacious therapeutic regimens that do not lend themselves to randomized, controlled trials. As a case in point, there may be patients who clearly would not benefit from CBT, but might benefit from interpersonal psychotherapy (IP) (39). Landers has noted that women in particular may derive positive benefits from IP. Blatt disavowed the notion that

CBT would be effective for all and charged clinicians to adapt the therapeutic approach both to the severity of the depression and the style best suited to particular patients (92). Furthermore, Blatt identified a type of depression that is intractable to short-term psychotherapy or medication, a severe type of depression based on a personality style of perfectionism. In further analyzing data from the NIMH Treatment of Depression Collaborative Research Program, a randomized, controlled trial of CBT, IP, medication, and placebo, Blatt et al. noted that, at 18-month follow-up, psychotherapy was more effective in improving interpersonal relationships and in creating an understanding about depression than were the medication and placebo groups (93). For some patients, then, Blatt postulates that long-term psychotherapy focusing on the development of an excellent therapeutic alliance with the patient and on an interpersonal approach to psychotherapy may be most effective. IP has also been demonstrated to assist recurrently depressed women in weathering life stressors and lengthening the time to recurrence of depression (94).

A multi-faceted approach to the treatment of depression is described in the accompanying table, known as the ASCEND model (Table 2). This model focuses on the subjective experience of the depressed patient of being in a "deep, dark hole" or "living life in a dark fog." Patients often describe their condition as being one that engenders a sense of working against heavy oppressive weights or having a difficult precipitous climb to accomplish any activities, however minor. They also feel "weighted down" and as if their thinking and emotive processes may be slow, non-functional, or muted. The treatment model focuses on several different aspects or strategies from different psychotherapeutic models and is one that primary care physicians can readily apply in a series of moderate length medical encounters. The strategy focuses on exercises and activities that patients complete between medical visits and attends to reinstituting activities or processes that the patient employed before the onset of depression.

The current discussion about treatment protocols emphasizes techniques that can be adopted by primary care physicians and applied in an ambulatory setting. Collaborative care, primary care physicians working with mental health specialists, is the ideal model, but it is important for physicians to understand effective treatments for psychological disorders, as well as to be able to conduct treatment in cases where patients decline referral to a mental health provider.

D. Pharmacotherapy in Perimenopausal Emotional Disorders

1. Antidepressants and Anxyolitics

Treatment with psychotropic medication should be reserved for patients with a diagnosed anxiety disorder or unipolar depression. Should the issue of prescribing a selective serotonin re-uptake inhibitor (SSRI), serotonin/norepinephrine re-uptake inhibitor (SNRI), or benzodiazepine arise in cases of uncertain diagnosis, the primary care provider may wish to consider referral for a psychiatric diagnostic interview to determine the presence of a specific anxiety disorder or clinical depression. Studies have demonstrated a benefit for pharmacological treatment of patients with anxiety and depression. The Depression Panel concluded that there is an A level of strength of evidence for treating moderate to severe major depressive disorder with medication, with randomized controlled trials documenting good efficacy for this group of depressed patients (95). Agents that affect both serotonin and norepinephrine may offer greater efficacy in terms of a stronger clinical response and less likelihood of relapse in depression (96). A meta-analysis of over 2000 patients in

Table 2 The ASCEND Model of the Primary Care Treatment of Depression

Activities
Sleep hygiene
Cognitive Behavioral Techniques
Exercise
Nurturance (self-support and social support)
Diet and **D**rug Therapy

1. Activities: Have the patient schedule activities that were formerly enjoyable, such as reading, talking, walking, dancing, church-going, or hobbies. Tell patients that "mood follows behavior" and if they resume their activities, their mood should elevate. They should structure time every day for some activities and on a weekly basis for others.
2. Sleep Hygiene: Have the patient follow the sleep program (Table 1). Tell them that this program should significantly improve their getting to sleep and staying asleep and that it has a higher long-term success rate than medication. Educate them that about 70% of patients in the peri/menopause have disordered sleep, that it is normal to have some problems, and that improvement requires patience and daily adherence to the program.
3. Cognitive Behavioral Techniques: Explain that if patients will change their thinking patterns, they can combat mood difficulties of depression and anxiety. Request that they develop a list of positive statements about themselves or life situations (affirmations). Two examples would be the statements, "I accept myself the way that I am" and "I work hard at what I do and others appreciate this." Then instruct them to substitute these positive thoughts for "automatic" negative thoughts. They can also replace troubling thoughts by visualizing a happier or calmer time or a powerful event, such as the birth of a child. Refer them to the self-care educational materials for depression and anxiety, such as Dr. Burn's Feeling Good Workbook and Dr. Bourne's Phobias and Anxiety Disorders Workbook.
4. Exercise: Tell the patient that research has shown that exercise is associated with lower rates of depression and anxiety and that 45 minutes of daily walking is the very best "cure" they can implement. Exercise also improves sleep. Let them know that perimenopausal women who exercise have lower levels of psychological distress.
5. Nurturance: Patients will benefit from supportive "self-talk" such as the affirmations and in completing activities that are self-nurturing, such as taking warm baths or reading their favorite uplifting texts. They also will benefit from support from others by letting friends/family members know they need some assistance or reassurance, or by participating in a support group or formal counseling. The primary care provider is crucial in offering appropriate professional support, encouragement, and nurturance to patients by regularly scheduled visits and by assuring them that treatment approaches can be successful.
6. Diet: Counsel patients about maintaining a balanced diet and reducing or avoiding stimulating or depressant substances, such as nicotine, caffeine, and alcohol.
   Drugs: Appropriately prescribe psychopharmacological agents for patients who meet DSM-IV criteria for an anxiety disorder or depression if the patient is amenable to this form of treatment. Target the two most significant symptoms of the disorder for each patient. Follow-up at 1, 3, 6, and 12 months to be certain that the targeted symptoms are positively affected by the medication or switch or add agents, if not. Counsel patients about expected side effects and encourage them to contact you if they have concerns. If agents are prescribed for sleep induction, consider having the patient use them no more than three nights per week, as this regimen offers significant improvement in sleep on some nights and adaptation or dependence is less likely to develop than a daily regimen.

international and U.S. studies documented that an agent that affects both serotonin and norepinephrine showed more efficacy after immediate treatment effects than an SSRI alone (97). The anxiety disorders, GAD, panic disorder, and social phobia, have been shown to be responsive to benzodiazepines (especially the higher potency ones) without significant risk of misuse in patients without a history of substance abuse (53). SSRIs are now often used as first line treatments for these anxiety disorders, with multiple agents being FDA approved for the treatment of GAD (venlafaxine, escitalopram, paroxetine and sertraline) (98,99).

2. Problems with SSRI Use

Physicians tend to see the selective serotonin re-uptake inhibitors as safe and highly effective medications. However, many patients are maintained on them for a significant period of time without careful re-evaluation by clinicians and may experience troubling side effects, some of which may ultimately exacerbate the original dysphoric state. One of the main issues in this regard is the anecdotal reporting of significant weight gain over longer-term treatment with the SSRIs. The high incidence of sexual dysfunction in both men and women has been well noted in the literature, including lowered levels of desire and anorgasmia. As ahedonia and loss of libido are two major criteria of depression, it is apparent that the potential remedy (an SSRI) can contribute to some of the very symptoms of the disorder it was designed to treat. Additionally, sudden withdrawal of short acting SSRIs may precipitate serotonin withdrawal syndrome, and patients must be cautioned against abrupt discontinuation of their medications. Interactions with other drugs may also occur. For example, SSRIs may not be used with MAO inhibitors, and patients should be specifically counseled to avoid the use of preparations of St. John's Wort while on SSRIs as the effects are synergistic. The antimicrobial linezolid may also increase serotonin levels and increase the risk for serotonin syndrome. Physicians now have at their disposal electronic databases that facilitate checking for drug to drug interactions (103).

E. Hormone Replacement Therapy and Psychological Symptoms

1. Use of HRT to Alter Psychological Symptoms

Controversy surrounds the role of hormone replacement therapy (HRT) in treating psychological symptoms and psychiatric conditions in the perimenopause. It is unclear if HRT directly improves psychological symptoms or indirectly impacts psychological symptoms by improving vasomotor and somatic symptoms related to the menopause transition (104). Some advocate a trial of HRT with close follow-up, especially if vasomotor and sleep disturbances are prominent (105,106). While the possible benefit of estrogen replacement on depressive symptoms has been hypothesized for years, the evidence is unclear for the perimenopausal period. The efficacy of the use of hormone replacement therapy as a synergistic agent to antidepressants in perimenopausal mood disorders is also unclear (107), although it is known that estrogen can alter serotonin receptors in postmenopausal women (108).

A meta-analysis of 38 studies employing HRT in menopausal women suggested that estrogen alone, or with the addition of androgen, was effective in reducing depressed mood, but progestins diminished the effect (109). Burt, Altshuler, and Rasgon, in reviewing studies focused on the association between depressive symptoms and the perimenopause, concluded that estrogen replacement may improve symptoms of lowered mood or dysphoria in perimenopausal patients without major unipolar depression (42). Further, they stated that there is no evidence to suggest that estrogen would offer any benefit as either a primary or adjunctive treatment for DSM-IV major depressive disorder during the perimenopause. Another study corroborates this idea of an improvement in some symptoms with mildly disordered mood. In a placebo-controlled, double-blind trial, 80% of women on estradiol replacement therapy had a full or partial improvement in depressive symptoms compared to 22% of those on placebo in a short trial of three to six weeks (110). Most of the women in this study had minor, rather than major depression, however, and the improvements were noted in some target symptoms of low mood and social isolation. Other symptoms—sleep disorder, hyperphagia and weight gain, fatigue, somatic symptoms, and feelings of unreality—did not change with estradiol. The type of sleep disorder women experience in peri- and postmenopause may be improved with estrogen replacement and progestogens may improve sleep-disordered breathing, which is not unique to estrogen deprivation (111). The 2007 position statement of NAMS acknowledged that a subgroup of women in the perimenopause may be at an increased risk of significant major depression. However, NAMS noted that there is insufficient evidence to support the general use of estrogen or estrogen and progestogen supplementation to treat depressive symptoms (2).

2. Increased Symptoms with HRT Use and with Surgical Menopause

Women who are treated with hormone replacement therapy (HRT) or who undergo a surgical menopause, however, appear to be different in their responses to the menopause transition than women who experience a natural menopause (4,6,112). Women with surgical menopause tend to have more noticeable emotional symptoms, as do women who are using HRT. It is unknown whether the underlying reason for surgery or HRT treatment confounds the picture in these women. In terms of HRT, it may be the effect of progestins, rather than estrogen, that is connected to the increase in symptoms. Bech and colleagues reported an improvement in psychological symptoms with both combined or sequential estrogen and progesterone treatment strategies in postmenopausal women as measured with Beck Depression Inventory and General Health Questionnaire (113). Girdler and colleagues reported greater anxiety symptoms, as well as depression, in women on combination estrogen and progesterone therapy in the progesterone treatment phase while patients on estrogen alone experienced no change in psychological symptoms (114). The increase in symptoms was not considered clinically significant, however. Interestingly, the placebo group experienced a robust reduction in irritability on rating scales. Other investigators advocate the use of natural progesterone in favor of synthetic progestins in order to avoid this phenomenon (115,116). An improvement in anxiety and depressive symptoms, as well as vasomotor complaints improved in one study for women on micronized natural progesterone as compared with medroxyprogesterone acetate (117). With the findings from the Women's Health Initiative, the role of HRT in caring for menopausal and perimenopausal women became more complex and controversial (118). The research indicated significant increased risks for some diseases (breast cancer and cardiovascular conditions) and decreased risks for osteoporosis and colon cancer. The potential benefits and risks for a particular patient must be weighed and all relevant factors (age, menopausal phase, risk of particular diseases) must be considered (2,119)."

IV. PATIENT EDUCATION

*A. What Patients Should Know About Psychological Disorders
   in the Perimenopause:*

- There are many myths about menopause and the years that proceed it (the perimenopause). It is always very difficult to ferret out the truth from "word of mouth" information, as well as to reasonably interpret the research literature about changes during this phase of life.

- There are two truths that can be unequivocally stated, one being that many women report very little noticeable change either physically, emotionally, or cognitively during the perimenopause. The second truth is that some women experience profound physical, emotional, or cognitive changes that are quite distressing and interfere with their usual functioning and these women present to health care providers for information and solutions to their difficulties. The vast majority of women likely fall between these points on a continuum and may experience a constellation of symptoms, with some types being more dominant for each individual than others. Just as women experienced their menstrual cycles quite differently from others, so too will be their experience of the perimenopause. In fact, it appears that women's symptoms during the premenstrual phase of their menstrual cycles may provide a clue to possible difficulties during the perimenopause.

*B. What Self-help Materials Are Available for Managing Mild to Moderate
   Symptoms of Depressed Mood or Anxiety?*

There are several excellent resources in this area: Dr. Burns' Feeling Good Workbook, Dr. Bourne's Phobia and Anxiety Workbook, and Dr. Miller's audiotapes or CDs, www.drmiller.com

C. What Professional Treatment Approaches Work Best for Anxiety and Depression?

Psychotherapy, including a type of treatment called cognitive behavior therapy, has been shown to significantly improve depression and anxiety with a limited number of counseling sessions. The active participation of women with one of these conditions in completing out-of-session assignments, such as using audiotapes and monitoring their thought processes that affect mood, is crucial to success. Other women profit from a different type of approach to therapy, called interpersonal psychotherapy. If couple discord or relationship issues seem to be the crux of the problem, then participation in couple counseling may be very beneficial.

*D. Should I Take Psychotropic Medications, Hormones or OTC Agents to
   Improve my Mood?*

Medications are a decision that must be made between a woman and her physician. The research shows that some women clearly benefit from both psychotropic medication and from hormone support in the perimenopause, while others show no benefit. Since all medications have some side effects, you should ask your health care provider about these and take this into consideration. OTC preparations also can have significant side effects, especially if they interact with prescription medications. Again, the best advice is to have a trusted health care provider who will discuss benefits and risks as you try to decide what is best for you.

REFERENCES

1. The North American Menopause Society. Clinical challenges of perimenopause: consensus opinion of the North American Menopause Society. Menopause: The Journal of the North American Menopause Society 2000; 7(1):5–13.
2. The North American Menopause Society. Estrogen and progestogen use in peri- and post-menopausal women: March 2007 position statement of The North American Menopause Society. Menopause: The Journal of the North American Menopause Society 2007; 14(2):168–182.
3. Avis NE, McKinlay SM. The Massachusetts Women's Health Study: an epidemiologic investigation of the menopause. J Am Med Womens Assoc 1995; 50(2):45–49.
4. Matthews KA, Wing RR, Kuller LH et al. Influences of natural menopause on psychological characteristics and symptoms of middle-aged healthy women. J Consult Clin Psychol 1990; 58(3):345–351.
5. Groeneveld FP, Bareman FP, Barentsen R et al. Vasomotor symptoms and well-being in the climacteric years. Maturitas 1996; 23(3):293–299.
6. Porter M, Penney GC, Russell D et al. A population-based survey of women's experience of the menopause. Br J Obstet Gynaecol 1996; 103(10):1025–1028.
7. Holte A, Mikkelsen A. Psychosocial determinants of climacteric complaints. Maturitas 1991; 13(3):205–215.
8. Rosenthal MB. Psychological aspects of menopause. Prim Care 1979; 6(2):357–364.
9. Woods NF, Mitchell ES. Pathways to depressed mood for midlife women: observations from the Seattle Midlife Women's Health Study. Res Nurs Health 1997; 20(2):119–129.
10. Ballinger CB. Psychiatric morbidity and the menopause; screening of general population sample. Br Med J 1975; 3(5979):344–346.
11. Avis NE, Stellato R, Crawford S et al. Is there a menopausal syndrome? Menopausal status and symptoms across racial/ethnic groups. Soc Sci Med 2001; 52:345–356.
12. Maartens LW, Leusink GL, Knottnerus JA. Climacteric complaints in the community. Fam Pract 2001; 18(2):189–194.
13. Sagsoz N, Oguzturk O, Bayram M et al. Anxiety and depression before and after the menopause. Arch Gynecol Obstet 2001; 264(4):199–202.
14. Dennerstein L, Dudley EC, Hopper JL et al. A prospective population-based study of menopausal symptoms. Obstet Gynecol 2000; 96(3):351–358.
15. Morse CA, Dudley E, Guthrie J et al. Relationships between premenstrual complaints and perimenopausal experiences. J Psychosom Obstet Gynaecol 1998; 19(4):182–191.
16. Daly E, Gray A, Barlow D et al. Measuring the impact of menopausal symptoms on quality of life. BMJ 1993; 307(6908):836–840.
17. Groeneveld FP, Bareman FP, Barensten R et al. The climacteric and well-being. J Psychosom Obstet Gynaecol 1993; 14(2):127–143.
18. Groeneveld FP, Bareman FP, Barensten R. Relationships between attitude towards menopause, well-being and medical attention among women aged 45–60 years. Maturitas 1993; 17(2):77–88.
19. Holte A. Influences of natural menopause on health complaints: a prospective study of healthy Norwegian women. Maturitas 1992; 14(2):127–141.
20. Kaufert PA, Gilbert P, Tate R. The Manitoba Project: a re-examination of the link between menopause and depression. Maturitas 1992; 14(2):143–155.
21. Stewart DE, Boydell K, Derzko C et al. Psychologic distress during the menopausal years in women attending a menopause clinic. Int J Psychiatry Med 1992; 22(3):213–220.
22. Hunter M, Battersby R, Whitehead M. Relationships between psychological symptoms, somatic complaints and menopausal status. Maturitas 1986; 8(3):217–228.
23. Cooke DJ. Social support and stressful life events during mid-life. Maturitas 1985; 7(4): 303–313.
24. Bromberger JT, Matthews KA. A longitudinal study of the effects of pessimism, trait anxiety, and life stress on depressive symptoms in middle-aged women. Psychol Aging 1996; 11(2):207–213.

25. Bromberger JT, Meyer PM, Kravitz HM et al. Psychologic distress and natural menopause: a multiethnic community study. Am J Public Health 2001; 91(9):1435–1442.

26. Greene JG, Hart DM. Evaluation of a psychological treatment programme for climacteric women. Maturitas 1987; 9(1):41–48.

27. Neri I, Demyttenaere K, Facchinetti F. Coping style and climacteric symptoms in a clinical sample of postmenopausal women. J Psychosom Obstet Gynaecol 1997; 18(3):229–233.

28. McKinlay SM, Brambilla DJ, Posner JG. The normal menopause transition. Maturitas 1992; 14(2):103–115.

29. Avis NE, Brambilla D, McKinlay SM et al. A longitudinal analysis of the association between menopause and depression. Results from the Massachusetts Women's Health Study. Ann Epidemiol 1994; 4(3):214–220.

30. Eaton WW, Kessler LG. Epidemiologic Field Methods in Psychiatry: The NIMH Epidemiologic Catchment Area Program. New York: Academic Press, Inc., 1985.

31. U.S. Dept. of Health and Human Services, National Institute of Mental Health. Epidemiologic Catchment Area Study, 1980–1985. Rockville, MD: U.S. Dept. of Health and Human Services, National Institute of Mental Health, 1992.

32. Blazer DG, Kessler RC, McGonagle KA et al. The prevalence and distribution of major depression in a national community sample: the National Comorbidity Survey. Am J Psychiatry 1994; 151(7):979–986.

32a. American Psychiatric Association. Diagnostic and Statistical Manual of Mental Disorders. 4th edn, Text Revision. Washington, DC: American Psychiatric Association, 2000.

33. Rodney J, Prior N, Cooper B et al. The comorbidity of anxiety and depression. Aust N Z J Psychiatry 1997; 31(5):700–703.

34. Beck AT, Steer RA, Ball R et al. Comparison of Beck Depression Inventories IA and II in psychiatric outpatients. J Pers Assess 1996; 67(3):588–597.

35. Zung WW. A self-rating depression scale. Arch Gen Psychiatry 1965; 12(1):63–70.

36. Zung WW. A rating instrument for anxiety disorders. Psychosomatics 1971; 12(6):371–379.

37. Turner JA, Romano JM. Self-report screening measures for depression in chronic pain patients. J Clin Psychol 1984; 40(4):909–913.

38. Shedler J, Beck A, Bensen S. Practical mental health assessment in primary care. Validity and utility of the Quick PsychoDiagnostics Panel. J Fam Pract 2000; 49(7):614–621.

39. Landers S. Both therapy, drugs, help with depression. The APA Monitor 1990; 21(2):25.

40. Robins LN, Helzer JE, Weissman MM et al. Lifetime prevalence of specific psychiatric disorders in three sites. Arch Gen Psychiatry 1984; 41(10):949–958.

41. Depression Guideline Panel. Depression in Primary Care: Volumes 1 and 2. Clinical Practice Guideline, Number 5. Rockville, MD. U.S. Department of Health and Human Services, Public Health Service, Agency for Health Care Policy and Research. AHCPR Publication No. 93–0550/1. April 1993.

42. Burt VK, Altshuler LL, Rasgon N. Depressive symptoms in the perimenopause: prevalence, assessment, and guidelines for treatment. Harv Rev Psychiatry 1998; 6(3):121–132.

43. Schmidt PJ, Roca CA, Bloch M et al. The perimenopause and affective disorders. Semin Reprod Endocrinol 1997; 15(1):91–100.

44. Busch CM, Zonderman AB, Costa PT. Menopausal transition and psychological distress in a nationally representative sample: Is menopause associated with psychological distress? J Aging Health 1994; 6(2):209–228.

45. Owens JF, Matthews KA. Sleep disturbance in healthy middle-aged women. Maturitas 1998; 30(1):41–50.

46. Baker A, Simpson S, Dawson D. Sleep disruption and mood changes associated with menopause. J Psychosom Res 1997; 43(4):359–369.

47. Shaver JL, Paulsen VM. Sleep, psychological distress, and somatic symptoms in perimenopausal women. Fam Pract Res J 1993; 13(4):373–384.

48. Li S, Holm K, Gulanick M et al. Perimenopause and the quality of life. Clin Nurs Res 2000; 9(1):6–23.

49. Kessler RC, McGonagle KA, Zhao S. Lifetime and 12-month prevalence of DSM III-R psychiatric disorders in the United States. Results from the National Comorbidity Survey. Arch Gen Psychiatry 1994; 51(1):8–19.

50. Boyd JH, Rae DS, Thompson JW et al. Phobia: prevalence and risk factors. Soc Psychiatry Psychiatr Epidemiol 1990; 25(6):314–323.

51. Wells JE, Bushnell JA, Hornblow AR et al. Christchurch Psychiatric Epidemiology Study, Part I: Methodology and lifetime prevalence for specific psychiatric disorders. Aust N Z J Psychiatry 1989; 23(3):315–326.

52. Tohen M, Bromet E, Murphy JM et al. Psychiatric epidemiology. Harv Rev Psychiatry 2000; 8(3):111–125.

53. Gorman JM. Anxiety disorders: clues to diagnosis, keys to therapy. Consultant 2001; 41(Suppl): S6–S12.

54. Regier DA, Rae DS, Narrow WE et al. Prevalence of anxiety disorders and their comorbidity with mood and addictive disorders. Br J Psychiatry Suppl 1998; 34:24–28.

55. Meyers JK, Weissman MM, Tischler GL et al. Six-month prevalence of psychiatric disorders in three communities 1980 to 1982. Arch Gen Psychiatry 1984; 41(10):959–967.

56. Birge SJ, McEwen BS, Wise PM. Effects of estrogen deficiency on brain function. Implications for the treatment of postmenopausal women. Postgrad Med 2001:11–16.

57. Robinson D, Friedman L, Marcus R et al. Estrogen replacement therapy and memory in older women. J Am Geriatr Soc 1994; 42(9):919–922.

58. Lichtman R. Perimenopausal and postmenopausal hormone replacement therapy. Part 2. Hormonal regimens and complementary and alternative therapies. J Nurse Midwifery 1996; 41(3):195–210.

59. Paganini-Hill A, Henderson VW. Estrogen deficiency and risk of Alzheimer's disease in women. Am J Epidemiol 1994; 140(3):256–261.

60. Fillit H. Estrogens in the pathogenesis and treatment of Alzheimer's disease in postmenopausal women. Ann NY Acad Sci 1994; 743: 233–238.

61. Mulnard RA, Cotman CW, Kawas C et al. Estrogen replacement therapy for treatment of mild to moderate Alzheimer's disease: A 1-year randomized controlled trial. Alzheimer's Disease Cooperative Study. JAMA 2000; 283(8):1007–1015.

61a. Shumaker SA, Legault C, Kuller L, et al. Conjugated equine estrogens and incidence of probable dementia and mild cognitive impairment in postmenopausal women: women's health initiative memory study. JAMA. 2004; 291:2947–2958.

62. Dennerstein L, Smith AM, Morse C et al. Menopausal symptoms in Australian women. Med J Aust 1993; 159(4):232–236.

63. Green JG. Psychosocial influences and life events at the time of the menopause. In: Formanek R, ed. The Meaning of Menopause: Historical, Medical and Clinical Perspectives. New Jersey: The Analytic Press, 1990:79–115.

64. McKinlay JB, McKinlay SM, Brambilla D. The relative contributions of endocrine changes and social circumstances to depression in mid-aged women. J Health Soc Behav 1987; 28(4):345–63.

65. Lock M. Ambiguities of aging: Japanese experience and perceptions of menopause. Cult Med Psychiatry 1986; 10(1):23–46.

66. Becker D, Lomranz J, Pines A et al. Psychological distress around menopause. Psychosomatics 2001; 42(3):252–257.

67. Burns DD. Feeling Good: The New Mood Therapy. New York: New American Library, 1980.

68. Burns DD. The Feeling Good Handbook. New York: Penguin Group, 1989.

69. Bourne EJ. The Anxiety and Phobia Workbook. 3rd edn. Oakland: New Harbinger Publications, 2000.

70. Greist JH, Jefferson JW, Marks IM. Anxiety and its Treatment: Help is Available. Washington DC: American Psychiatric Press, 1986.

71. Beck AT, Emery G. Anxiety Disorders and Phobias: A Cognitive Perspective. New York: Basic Books, 1985.

72. Garry J, Whetstone L. Physical activity and exercise at menopause. Clin Fam Prac 2002; 4:1–19.
73. Miszko TA, Cress ME. A lifetime of fitness. Exercise in the perimenopausal and postmeno-pausal woman. Clin Sports Med 2000; 19(2):215–232.
74. Slaven L, Lee C. Mood and symptom reporting among middle-aged women: the relationship between menopausal status, hormone replacement therapy, and exercise participation. Health Psychol 1997; 16(3):203–208.
75. Kosch SG, Burg MA, Podikuju S. Patient ethnicity and diagnosis of emotional disorders in women. Fam Med 1998; 30(3):215–219.
76. Babyak M, Blumenthal JA, Herman S et al. Exercise treatment for major depression: maintenance of therapeutic benefit at 10 months. Psychosom Med 2000; 62(5):633–638.
77. Blumenthal JA, Babyak MA, Moore KA et al. Effects of exercise training on older patients with major depression. Arch Intern Med 1999; 159(19):2349–2356.
78. Morin CM, Kwentus JA. Behavioral and pharmacological treatments for insomnia. Annals Behav Med 1988; 10:91–100.
79. Bootzin RR, Rider SP. Behavioral techniques and biofeedback for insomnia. In: Pressman MR, Orr WC, eds. Understanding Sleep: The Evaluation and Treatment of Sleep Disorders. Application and Practice in Health Psychology. Washington DC: American Psychological Association, 1997:315–338.
80. Bootzin R, Nicassio P. Behavioral treatments of insomnia. In: Hensen M, Eisler R, Miller P, eds. Progress in Behavior Modification. New York: Academic Press, 1978:1–45.
81. Anarte MT, Cuadros JL, Herrera J. Hormonal and psychological treatment: therapeutic alternative for menopausal women? Maturitas 1998; 29(3):203–213.
82. Beck AT, Rush AJ, Shaw BF et al. Cognitive Therapy of Depression. New York: Guilford Press, 1979.
83. Teasdale JD, Moore RG, Hayhurst H et al. Metacognitive awareness and prevention of relapse in depression: empirical evidence. J Consult Clin Psychol 2002; 70(2):275–287.
84. Wells KB, Sherbourne C, Schoenbaum M et al. Impact of disseminating quality improvement programs for depression in managed primary care: a randomized controlled trial. JAMA 2000; 283(2):212–220.
85. Gordon VC, Matwychuk AK, Sachs EG et al. A 3-year follow-up of a cognitive behavioral therapy intervention. Arch Psychiatr Nurs 1988; 2(4):218–226.
86. Norman J, Lowry CE. Evaluating inipatient treatment for women with clinical depression. Res Social Work Prac 1995; 5(1):10–19.
87. Newman MG, Borkovec TD. Cognitive behavioral treatment of generalized anxiety disorder. The Clin Psychologist 1995; 48(4):5–7.
88. Durham RC, Murphy T, Allan T et al. Cognitive therapy, analytic psychotherapy and anxiety management training for generalized anxiety disorder. Br J Psychiatry 1994; 165(3):315–323.
89. Fava GA, Rafanelli C, Grandi S et al. Prevention of recurrent depression with cognitive behavioral therapy: preliminary findings. Arch Gen Psychiatry 1998; 55(9):816–820.
90. Derubeis RJ. Advances in the treatment of depression. American Psychological Association 110th Annual Convention, Chicago, Illinois, August 23, 2002.
91. Holmes, J. All you need is cognitive behaviour therapy? BMJ 2002; 324(7332):288–290.
92. Blatt SJ. The destructiveness of perfectionism. Implications for the treatment of depression. Am Psychol 1995; 50(12):1003–1020.
93. Blatt SJ, Zuroff DC, Bondi CM et al. Short- and long-term effects of medication and psychotherapy in the brief treatment of depression: further analyses of data from the NIMH TDCRP. Psychother Res 2000; 10(2):215–234.
94. Harkness KL, Frank E, Anderson B. Does interpersonal psychotherapy protect women from depression in the face of stressful life events? J Consult Clin Psychol 2002;70(4):908–915.
95. Kelsey JE. Treating depression: beyond response to remission. Consultant 2001; 4 (Suppl): S13–S19.
96. Clerc GE, Ruimy P, Verdeau-Palles J. A double-blind comparison of venlafaxine and fluoxetine in patients hospitalized for a major depression and melancholia. The Venlafaxine French Inpatient Study Group. Int Clin Psychopharmacol 1994; 9(3):139–143.

97. Thase ME, Entsuah AR, Rudolph RL. Remission rates during treatment with venlafaxine or selective serotonin reuptake inhibitors. Br J Psychiatry 2001; 178:234–241.

98. Pollack MH, Zaninelli R, Goddard A et al. Paroxetine in the treatment of generalized anxiety disorder: results of a placebo-controlled, flexible dosage trial. J Clin Psychiatry 2001; 62(5):350–357.

99. Gelenberg AJ, Lydiard RB, Rudolph RL et al. Efficacy of venlafaxine extended-release capsules in nondepressed outpatients with generalized anxiety disorder: A 6-month randomized controlled trial. JAMA 2000; 283(23):3082–3088.

100. Stahl SM. Natural estrogen as an antidepressant for women. J Clin Psychiatry 2001; 62(6): 404–405.

101. Hypericum Depression Trial Study Group. Effect of Hypericum perforatum (St. John's wort) in major depressive disorder: a randomized controlled trial. JAMA 2002; 287(14):1807–1814.

102. Behnke K, Jensen GS, Graubaum HJ et al. Hypericum perforatum versus fluoxetine in the treatment of mild to moderate depression. Adv Ther 2002; 19(1):43–52.

103. Gaster B, Holroyd J. St. John's wort for depression: a systematic review. Arch Intern Med 2000; 160(2):152–156.

104. Alder EM, Ross LA, Gebbic A. Menopausal symptoms and the domino effect. J Reprod Infant Psychol 2000; 18(1):75–78.

105. Boyle GJ, Murrihy R. A preliminary study of hormone replacement therapy and psychological mood states in perimenopausal women. Psychol Rep 2001; 88(1):160–170.

106. Consensus Opinion. Clinical challenges of perimenopause: consensus opinion of the North American Menopause Society. Menopause 2000; 7(1):5–13.

107. Stahl SM. Augmentation of antidepressants by estrogen. Psychopharmacol Bull 1998; 34(3):319–321.

108. Halbreich U, Rojansky N, Palter S. Estrogen augments serotonergic activity in postmenopausal women. Biol Psychiatry 1993; 37:434–441.

109. Zweifel JE, O'Brien WH. A meta-analysis of the effect of hormone replacement therapy upon depressed mood. Psychoneuroendocrinology 1997; 22(3):189–212

110. Schmidt PJ, Nieman L, Danaceau MA et al. Estrogen replacement in perimenopause-related depression: a preliminary report. Am J Obstet Gynecol 2000; 183(2):414–420.

111. Polo-Kantola P, Saaresranta T, Polo O. Aetiology and treatment of sleep disturbances during perimenopause and postmenopause. CNS Drugs 2001; 15(6):445–452.

112. Kuh DL, Wadsworth M, Hardy R. Women's health in midlife: the influence of the menopause, social factors and health in earlier life. Br J Obstet Gynaecol 1997; 104(8):923–933.

113. Bech P, Munk-Jensen N, Obel EB et al. Combined versus sequential hormonal replacement therapy: a double-blind, placebo-controlled study on quality of life-related outcome measures. Psychother Psychosom 1998; 67(4–5):259–265.

114. Girdler SS, O'Briant C, Steege J et al. A comparison of the effect of estrogen with or without progesterone on mood and physical symptoms in postmenopausal women. J Womens Health Gend Based Med 1999; 8(5):637–646.

115. Vliet EL. Menopause and perimenopause: the role of ovarian hormones in common neuroendocrine syndromes in primary care. Prim Care 2002; 29(1):43–67.

116. Martorano JT, Ahlgrimm M, Colbert T. Differentiating between natural progesterone and synthetic progestins: clinical implications for premenstrual syndrome and perimenopause management. Compr Ther 1998; 24(6–7):336–339.

117. Fitzpatrick LA, Pace C, Wiita B. Comparison of regimens containing oral micronized progesterone or medoxyprogesterone acetate on quality of life in postmenopausal women: a cross-sectional survey. J Women's Health Gend Based Med 2000; 9(4):381–387.

118. Writing Group for the Women's Health Initiative Investigators. Risks and benefits of estrogen plus progestin in healthy postmenopausal women: principle results from the Women's Health Initiative randomized controlled trial. JAMA 2002; 288(3):321–333.

119. Fletcher SW, Colditz GA. Failure of estrogen plus progestin therapy for prevention. JAMA 2002; 288(3):366–368.

7

Sexuality of the Perimenopausal Patient

Shae Graham Kosch
Behavioral Medicine Program, Department of Community Health and Family Medicine, University of Florida College of Medicine, Gainesville, Florida, U.S.A.

I. INTRODUCTION

Over the last several decades, there has been an increase in research and treatment programs centered on women's sexual functioning and sexual dysfunctions. Until the 1970s, there were not many sex education materials available to the general public and there was a gap in scientific inquiry between the survey work of Kinsey and colleagues in the late 1940s and the more modern clinical and research efforts. An extensive body of literature on female sexual responding and dysfunction now exists and a variety of health care providers offer women effective treatment strategies to assist with particular problems.

The perimenopausal phase of life involves some alteration in physiological and psychosocial processes for all women. Peterson and Schmidt, in a longitudinal, prospective project of women aged 20 to 80, noted several changes specific to the perimenopausal period, including in serum levels of alkaline phosphatate, phosphorous, thyroxine, sleep patterns, and sexual functioning (1). As noted by Sulak, the major changes connected to ovarian failure are menstrual changes and vasomotor symptoms, which are experienced by most all perimenopausal women; other symptoms of significance include urogenital atrophy, infertility, declining bone mass, increased risk of heart disease, and psychosexual dysfunction (2). The following discussion focuses on sexual functioning in women, changes that occur with perimenopause and assessment and management approaches.

A. Research on Normal Female Sexual Response

In the 1960s and 1970s, efforts were directed toward delineating the physiological and psychological processes in women's sexual arousal and orgasm (3–5) and describing how societal and women's sexual attitudes affected behavior and functioning (6). This body of research and publications discredited many myths about female sexual functioning and helped clarify the role of hormonal, physiological, and psychological factors in healthy sexual functioning. First, for instance, therapists who focused on changing specific sexual behaviors—behavioral sex therapists—discounted the notion that all psychosexual dysfunction was the result of deep-seated intrapsychic or interpersonal processes that could be ameliorated solely by long-term analytic psychotherapy. Second, prior to some of this research, both health professionals and laypersons assumed that the major physical structure involved in the female orgasm was the vagina and that vaginal penetration was necessary for orgasm. The laboratory investigations of Masters and Johnson empirically demonstrated that this was untrue. The comprehensive work of Kaplan offered the clearest description of the process, detailing the fact that the sensory component involved in women's orgasmic responding is the clitoral body, while the circumvaginal muscles comprise the efferent aspect of the female orgasm (5). The clarification of these processes prompted behavioral sex therapists to develop constructive suggestions for women with orgasmic difficulties. Therapists recommended that couples adapt their sexual practices and techniques to address the sensory component involved in female sexual arousal, which should thus increase the ease of eliciting orgasm. Masters and Johnson identified four major phases of human sexual responding: excitement, plateau, orgasm, and resolution. Kaplan described three major patterns to female orgasm. The first pattern consists of a slow level of arousal, then reaching high plateau levels of responding with a minor orgasmic response, and then moving into resolution. The second would involve a more precipitous climb from arousal through plateau to a single relatively intense orgasm and into resolution. This pattern is one that more closely simulates the male sexual response pattern and research has shown that it is often experienced by women during non-coital activities. The third major pattern for women involves that of multiple orgasmic episodes and the researchers note that, since there is not a refractory period in the female orgasmic response as there is for males, additional orgasms after the first do not require that the woman return to baseline levels of arousal before a second orgasmic episode. (Helen Singer Kaplan provides a diagram of the different types of human response patterns that clinicians can use to clarify the patterns to patients.) The research also identified the type of psychosexual activities that women find most arousing and emphasized the importance of a lengthy foreplay period. For instance, it is important to note that women who are reliably orgasmic through coitus often participate in 20 to 25 minutes of foreplay with their partners prior to commencing intercourse. Scientific inquiry thus highlighted an important gender difference: Researchers noted that for males, especially younger ones, a briefer time of foreplay is adequate to create plateau levels of arousal to have men move from plateau to orgasmic responses, whereas for women a more lengthy excitement or arousal phase is required for them to progress satisfactorily through all four phases of sexual response.

Any current discussion of sexual functioning must acknowledge that most research projects or treatment protocols for sexual dysfunctions adhere to a traditional, biomedical approach that "medicalize" certain aspects of women's sexuality (7) and often extrapolate from male sexual functioning to that of women. The biomedical model has been critiqued and it has been noted that sexual interest and responding in women cannot be extrapolated from men's behavior. More global relationship factors, as well as a broader array of human interactions, are especially salient when evaluating women's sexual desire and interactions and constitute a "new view" of women's sexual problems (8). The following discussion focuses on traditional medical and psychological aspects of diagnosing and treating sexual dysfunction in women during the perimenopause, but also describes some important life experiences and their impact on the sexual functioning of women. Perimenopausal women often undergo significant changes in social situations and attitudes—these factors are frequently related to their sense of themselves as healthy or dysfunctional sexual beings.

B. Frequency of Sexual Dysfunctions

General medical outpatients frequently report sexual dysfunctions to health care providers if the clinicians elicit a comprehensive history and inquire about sexual function. Read, King and Watson report that 42% of women primary care patients report sexual dysfunction, while 68% report general sexual dissatisfaction (9). The rate of the particular sexual dysfunctions among these primary care patients was 30% for vaginismus and 23% for anorgasmia. Approximately 30% of women have a low level of desire and 25% are nonorgasmic (10). Other reports have noted that 14% to 50% have problems with arousal and plateau phases of the sexual response cycle. Although the incidence of sexual problems in both men and women is reportedly high, the incidence of true sexual dysfunction is lower when more stringent criteria are applied (11). In the U.S. culture, most heterosexual men and women believe that intercourse is one of the most important aspects of a good sexual relationship and that it is crucial for a woman to be comfortable during coitus and enjoy the activity. Sexual dysfunction can significantly affect a woman's quality of life and the interpersonal relationship with her partner(s). In terms of perimenopausal women, physiological changes occurring during this life phase can create barriers to comfortable, pleasurable coition and can reduce both sexual interest and ease of arousal.

C. Classification of Sexual Dysfunctions

The Consensus Development Panel on Female Sexual Dysfunction was established by the Sexual Function Health Council of the American Foundation for Urologic Disease and led to the development of a new classification system for the dysfunctions (12). All of the disorders are subclassified along three dimensions: (A) lifelong or acquired, (B) generalized or situational, and (C) etiology, including organic, psychogenic, mixed, or unknown. A complete evaluation of a potential sexual dysfunction would include a thorough history of the sexual problems, a physical and gynecological examination, and, certainly in perimenopausal women, an evaluation of hormonal status.

1. Sexual Desire Disorder

Definition: A woman who has personal distress about her low level of interest in sex or sexual activity and few or no sexual thoughts or fantasies. A disorder of desire involves the seeming inability of a woman to be aroused by what many or most would find to be pleasurable sexual activities. Some women appear to have a low level of desire throughout the life cycle; while others clearly experience decreases during periods of hormonal transitions or difficulties in personal relationships. Clearly, estrogen, progesterone, and testosterone all play pivotal roles in sexual functioning and sex hormone deprivation can profoundly affect libido, sexual fantasies, and urges, and the ability to experience early stages of sexual arousal. The most extreme disorder of desire is sexual aversion disorder, wherein a woman is distressed by her persistent aversion to or avoidance of sexual contact with a partner. This is one of the more difficult sexual problems to treat, and in the perimenopausal period, the problem may be correlated with a decline in gonadal hormones.

2. Sexual Arousal Disorder

Definition: A woman who is distressed by a persistent inability to obtain or maintain a sufficient sexual excitement during sexual activities, including self-perceived psychological arousal or somatic responses, such as vaginal lubrication and vasocongestion. Problems with arousal can be related to dysfunctions in the intrapsychic, interpersonal, or organic spheres. Women who have significant emotional inhibitions about sex, such as ones acquired during a restrictive or very religious childhood, often cannot maintain a state of psychological relaxation during sexual activities and may block the normal transmission of sensory impulses from erogenous zones (breasts, genitalia) to brain. Likewise, those who are ambivalent about their relationship with their partner or are in an interpersonally troubled relationship may be distracted by emotional issues and unable to focus on sexual responses and potential pleasure. Clearly, there are necessary hormonal substrates for physiological sexual arousal and adequate arousal is difficult to maintain in their absence.

3. Orgasmic Disorder

Definition: A woman who is personally distressed by a persistent/recurrent absence of orgasm or has delayed orgasm with adequate sexual arousal and adequate stimulation. Anorgasmia refers to the inability of a woman to attain orgasmic responding. It can be either primary, anorgasmia in a woman who has never been orgasmic; secondary, the inability to reach orgasm in a woman who was previously orgasmic; or situational, in which a woman may be able to attain orgasm with some activities or in some situations but not in others. Behavioral sex therapy is quite effective in teaching previously non-orgasmic women how to attain orgasm. Heiman and colleagues outlined a behavioral counseling program for primary anorgasmia that is highly effective, with treatment successes reported by different authors being in the 80% to 90% range (12). The program involves educating women about female anatomy and elements of the sexual response cycle; exploring attitudes toward sexual matters or activities that may serve as barriers to functioning; decreasing psychological inhibitions or embarrassment; encouraging the woman and her partner to explore sensory avenues for arousal; having the woman become an expert on what techniques are most effective in eliciting orgasm for her; and teaching her partner these techniques. For women who have situational dysfunction, who are orgasmic with direct or indirect stimulation of the clitoral body but are not orgasmic through intercourse, a behavioral program that pairs effective stimulatory techniques with intercourse can improve orgasmic response during coitus in many patients. One aspect that physicians should remember is that a woman's not being orgasmic through intercourse is a normal variant in the United States, as studies have identified 30% to 50% of women as having this variant. In a study of women seeing primary care physicians for their general health care (9), approximately 20% of women report difficulties with orgasm.

4. Sexual Pain Disorder

Definition of Sexual Pain Disorder: A woman who has recurrent/persistent pelvic or genital pain. This is subdivided into two types, vaginismus, in which a woman has pain with penetration and non-coital sexual pain disorder, in which a woman has recurrent/persistent pain during non-insertive activities. A woman who has a sexual dysfunction secondary to dyspareunia may have normal libido and normal sexual response cycles. Her functioning may only be impaired during particular activities (e.g., penetration) in which pain blocks any possible pleasurable responses, thus stopping the progression through the usual phases of the sexual response cycle. In addressing sexual dysfunction in the perimenopause, dyspareunia is a very important aspect to consider, as atrophic vaginitis is a major cause of pain during intercourse.

Vaginismus is usually defined as a situation wherein a woman has involuntary contractions of the circumvaginal muscles whenever an attempt at penetration occurs. As per the classification scheme, this may be a primary condition—with the woman having this dysfunction from the very first time that penetration is attempted—or it can be a secondary phenomenon; for instance, secondary to dyspareunia caused by pain first related to a herpes outbreak. A behavioral treatment approach can often be very effective in combating vaginismus and descriptions in Kaplan would assist any clinician trying to explain to a patient what the behavioral sex therapy approach would entail. One other important etiology to consider is the possibility that the vaginismus is due to dyspareunia associated with vulvar vestibulitis syndrome. This diagnostic condition requires a coordinated approach between a physician and a psychotherapist to assure that appropriate medications to anesthetize the vaginal vault are used, along with progressive dilation and other aspects of behavioral sex therapy. In the perimenopasual phase, vaginismus can develop secondary to dyspareunia related to lowered lubrication and increased vaginal tissue friability. Binik et al. suggest that the pain associated with vaginismus may not involve vaginal spasm and object to the "psychologizing" of what they view as a nonsexual pain disorder (13).

II. SEXUALITY IN THE PERIMENOPAUSE

A. Perimenopausal Changes and Sexual Functioning

Lowered levels of sex steroids and other physical alterations in women aged 40 to 55 create an increased likelihood of sexual difficulties. Psychological and interpersonal changes in the perimenopause may also clearly contribute to lowered interest or libido. The hallmark changes associated with the climacteric phase of life directly or indirectly can affect sexuality. As aptly and succinctly stated by Masters and Johnson: "A woman previously experiencing a healthy libido may become relatively asexual while contending with such menopausal discomforts as excessive fatigue, flushing, nervousness, emotional irritability, occipital headaches, or vague pelvic pain." (p. 242). Since many of these symptoms of the climacteric transition begin during the perimenopause, these also may constitute barriers to a woman's libidinous life during that phase. As Bachmann pointed out, many women who present to the gynecologist during the early years of perimenopause may complain of very distressing symptoms such as insomnia, menstrual difficulties, hot flashes, or mood swings and may not focus on sexual difficulties (14). However, if questioned about their sexual functioning, they may well report problematic changes. However, as Berman et al. emphasized, with 30% to 50% of the general population of American adult women experiencing sexual dysfunction, it is difficult to ascertain changes in the rates specific to the perimenopause or menopause (15).

As noted by Bachmann, most information about women's sexual functioning in the perimenopause are based on questionnaire data rather than laboratory measures of physiological and anatomical responding that are then correlated with hormonal data. There have been some perimenopause studies that incorporated more objective parameters and scientists have documented sexuality-related changes that occur both with age and with menopausal status. As Nachtigall emphasized, the symptoms of perimenopause are highly variable and difficult to measure (16). Levels of LH, FSH, and estradiol are inconsistent across women during the perimenopause, thus are of limited clinical value and cannot be reliably used to diagnose perimenopause. The only practical use of these assays has to do with FSH and fertility—a FSH level below 20 mIU/ml constitutes a risk of pregnancy, with that occurrence being less likely between 20 and 30 mIU/ml. IF the FSH is greater than 30 mIU/ml, pregnancy is not possible as this indicates that the ovaries are menopausal.

Berman et al. suggested assessing changes in women at various ages by using physiological measurements to evaluate organic dysfunction, such as the peak systolic velocity in the genitals, the pH of the vagina, intravaginal pressure-volume changes, and vibratory sensation thresholds in the vagina. Their research documented that both an older group of women aged 55 to 71 and menopausal women who were not hormone-replaced had significantly lower physiologic responses. This reduced functioning and increased sexual complaints, including low arousal, 67%; low desire, 21%; difficulty achieving orgasm, 92%; and pain or dyspareunia during or following intercourse, 67%. Obviously, the degree of dysfunction is considerably less in women aged 40 to 55, but both age and hormonal transitions begin the process of a decline in usual functioning. In general, research has shown that perimenopausal and menopausal women decrease the frequency of sexual activity and increase the severity of sexual dysfunction as they age. There is a generalized decrease in libido related to both lowered activity and dysfunction and this can especially affect certain aspects of the response cycle. In terms of specific genital changes, urogenital atrophy develops as hormonal stimulation of cells decrease. In the perimenopause, there is a thinning of the vaginal squamous epithelium and the vaginal vault becomes shorter, narrower, and less elastic, with a smoother surface, decrease in rugae, and lessened secretions (17).

B. Perimenopausal Changes and the Sexual Response Cycle

Cataloguing potential sexual problems by the affected phase of the sexual response cycle may best clarify the situation of perimenopausal changes.

1. Excitement Phase
- Lowered libido
- Decrease in sensitivity of the clitoral body
- Inadequate lubrication with sexual arousal
- Slower responding
- Requirement for longer or more intense sexual stimulation to achieve lubrication

2. Plateau Phase
- Inadequate vaginal lubrication
- Initiation of atrophy of vaginal vault
- Dyspareunia with penetration

3. Orgasmic Phase
- Decrease in sensitivity of the clitoral body
- Decreased frequency of orgasm with coitus
- Less intense orgasmic response
- Fewer contractions of the orgasmic platform at 0.8 seconds
- Diminishing/ lack of uterine contractions or potentially painful contractions

In regard to the changes in the orgasmic phase, Masters and Johnson noted that in younger women there are contractions of the pubococcygeal muscles at 0.8 seconds per minute which last for eight to ten contractions, while in the postmenopausal woman, these are reduced to three or four contractions. For perimenopausal women, the response may fall between these two parameters, with the result of a perceived lessening of the orgasmic response. The phenomenon of *status orgasmus* (a spasm of the circumvaginal muscles of two to four seconds preceding orgasmic contractions that can occur in some women during prolonged coition) does not occur in women as they move into their 40s.

C. Sociocultural Factors

It is difficult to ferret out the influence of social, psychological, interpersonal, and biological factors contributing to sexual changes or dysfunction in the perimenopause. Although it has been assumed that changes in hormonal status are directly responsible for changes in sexual functioning during the perimenopause and menopause, it is also important to consider social and psychological factors that may relate to the maintenance of a healthy sexual life. The United States has become an increasingly youth-focused culture and the beginnings of noticeable aging that occur during the perimenopause can be quite psychologically stressful to many women. Interpersonal factors are also important in terms of the quality of the affectionate life in a partnered relationship and the stability of the couple's relationship. There is no substitute for an affirming, positive partner in assuring a woman that she is attractive and sexually desirable. Many of the dilemmas or sexual impasses that women may experience during the climacteric period can be definitely ameliorated by the love and support of a sensitive and verbally caring partner. A positive love relationship was reported to be an essential ingredient in preserving a positive sexual functioning in the perimenopause and beyond (18). Certainly, altered body image is a major variable in women's sexual lives during the perimenopause. Notable physical changes related to this include skin laxity and/or wrinkling (19), a thickening of the waistline, and a relative decrease in muscle tone, loss of collagen tissue, which relates to changes in breast shape. These alterations that occur over the perimenopause into the menopausal period may prompt many women to feel self-conscious about their bodies and reduce their comfort in sexual activities, which then leads to an inhibition of natural response.

In a Danish study of 500 women interviewed at ages 40, 45, and 51, 70% had no change in sexual desire during those years. Current and previous levels of libido were associated with overall health status, social status, and partner availability. Anticipation of decreased libido with menopause was predictive of a decrease in libido (20). A study cited by Lichtman stated that of 2000 randomly surveyed women between 45 and 55, the majority reported no change in libido and when lowered libido was present, it was also associated with decreased well-being, employment status, and other symptomatology. Avis et al. reported on the 200 women in the Massachusetts Women's Health Study II, a population-based sample of women transitioning through natural menopause and not using HRT, and measured sexual functioning in terms of several variables (21). Overall, the findings from this project emphasize the multifactorial nature of sexual changes in the perimenopause. Menopausal status was significantly related to decreased libido, a psychosocial belief system positing that interest in sex declines over the life cycle, and a perceived decrease in perceived arousal compared to earlier in life. In regression analyses, other factors such as general health status, relationship status, mental health status, and smoking had a greater impact on women's sexual functioning than did menopausal status. In this study then, lifestyle variables were more powerful than hormonal status in determining sexual functioning in the climacteric.

D. Pregnancy in the Perimenopause

The perimenopausal years do not end concerns of unintended pregnancy and issues around conception and contraception can contribute to sexual problems. When vaginal dryness or frank dyspareunia exists, barrier methods of contraception are clearly more difficult to employ and can contribute to discomfort and pain. Also, many women (and their partners) in this age group are concerned about not bearing children, as evidenced by many unplanned pregnancies in women above the age of 40 being terminated by abortion (22); this group has the highest abortion rate next to teenagers (23). On the other hand, Masters and Johnson describe the concept that some women clearly experience an increased interest in sexual activity in the perimenopause. One phenomenon they observed was connected to women's desire to become pregnant before it becomes physiologically impossible, which may not represent an increased interest in sexual activities themselves, only a drive toward procreation. The second phenomenon, however, is related to a renewed interest or greater comfort with sex due to the lifting of a "pregnancy phobia" when contraception is no longer possible. Especially for women who have employed barrier methods to prevent contraception, when definite infertility arrives, there can be a sense of liberation from pregnancy concerns that leads to greater relaxation, spontaneity, and comfort with sexual relations.

III. HORMONAL STATUS AND SEXUAL FUNCTIONING

In direct opposition to the findings of the previously described studies, data from the Melbourne Women's Mid-life Health Project (24) showed that, as women completed the hormonal transitions from perimenopause through menopause, a decline in sexual interest was associated with hormonal status rather than a general decrease in well-being, educational level, employment outside the home, or higher levels of other symptoms. The role of hormonal status appears to be one that directly affects sexual functioning in the perimenopause. Some researchers have controlled potential confounding variables by studying women without serious medical illness and with a consistent, ongoing partner (25,26). The major findings of these series of projects have demonstrated that decreases in ovarian hormones are undisputedly related to a lowering of sexual functioning. Sarrel noted that hormones have various effects on the entire nervous system (27). For instance, the effects of androgens in the brain are mediated through androgen-specific receptors and by the aromatization of testosterone to estradiol and can play an important role in both psychological and sexual changes occurring during peri- and postmenopause. Another project (28) examined the relationships between premenopausal and postmenopausal symptoms, including obesity and attitudes toward sexuality, and other serum assays, that is glucose, cortisol, FSH, and prolactin. Symptoms included changes in sleep patterns and dysphoria and it was found that attitudes toward sexuality were associated with most menopausal symptoms.

One avenue of discussion in the literature focuses on the fact that the aging process, as well as hormonal changes, can influence women's sexual functioning. Hawton et al. noted an age-related pattern of incremental decline in the frequency of sexual intercourse in mid-life (29). Dennerstein, Dudley, and Burger designed a series of studies that examined women at various ages (38, 46, 50, 54) during active hormonal transitions and evaluated changes in sexual functioning as related to both age and hormonal status. By using a longitudinal study design of general population women and employing a validated rating scale that examined different aspects of sexual functioning (their relationship with their partner, sexual responsiveness, sexual activity level, libido, vaginal dryness, and dyspareunia), the authors were able to compare the relative effects of age and hormonal status. One finding of their series of projects noted that 62% of women aged 45 to 55 reported no change of sexual interest, 31% reported a decrease, and 7% reported an increase. Other data suggested that the only significant change in sexual functioning from early to late perimenopause was a change in sexual responsiveness, consisting of three aspects: arousal during sexual activities, enjoyment of those activities, and orgasm.

A. Estrogen

As estrogen declines, the vaginal vault exhibits clear changes in blood flow, pH levels, and secretory activity. The perimenopause does not lead to frank vaginal atrophy, but there are sufficient changes in the vaginal barrel that can make tactile sensitivity higher and can lead to dyspareunia with penetration if vaginal lubricants are not used on a regular basis before penetration. Significant non-vaginal changes due to estrogen decrease have also been described, especially changes in sensory perception, including signs suggestive of peripheral neuropathy with increased numbness or itching and potential aversion to touch. Lichtman further noted that there are effects of estrogen on the central and peripheral nervous symptoms, including vibration sense and on the cardiovascular system with effects on arterial blood flow. At the most serious end of the continuum, these types of changes might prompt a woman to be adverse to any skin touching or sexual interaction. One other important area of change with age/estrogen deficit involves the urinary tract. The research documents a benefit of estrogen replacement on reducing the number of urinary tract infections and urge incontinence and as inconclusive in affecting stress incontinence, sexual functioning unrelated to physical symptoms, and emotional symptoms (19).

Bachmann points out that women may not recognize their decrease in vaginal lubrication during sexual activities as being related to the early signs of estrogen decrease and may attribute psychosocial causes to this phenomenon. It is important to educate women carefully about expected changes due to hormonal aspects of the perimenopause so that they do not make incorrect assumptions. The same point certainly also applies to the nongenital changes noted above. Bachmann describes a vaginal health index developed at Robert Wood Johnson Medical School that details the overall elasticity of the vaginal vault, the type and consistency of fluid secretion, the pH, and the appearance and pliability of the epithelial mucosa. Bachmann also contends that estrogen replacement with low-dose oral contraceptives in the perimenopausal period may reverse many of the vaginal effects of estrogen decline. Studies by Semmens and Wagner detailed that estrogen replacement in women who had had bilateral ovariectomy had an impact on the entire sexual response cycle including the vasocongestion of the external genitalia and lower third of the vagina, clitoral responsiveness and engorgement, vaginal lubrication, the change in the length of the vaginal vault, and the contraction and elevation of the orgasmic platform and uterus (30). Estrogen replacement also normalized the vaginal pH to near 4.6 or below. According to Lichtman estrogen has been shown to be related to adequate vaginal lubrication, blood flow, appropriate thickness of the vaginal walls, and normal vaginal pH. The decrease in estrogen leads to a thinning of the vaginal walls and vaginal wall pliability, with concomitant irritation on contact, susceptibility to infection, and dyspareunia. Both systemic and local estrogen preparations are effective in reversing these symptoms.

The above reports clearly demonstrated a connection between estrogen deficit in the perimenopause and improvement in sexual functioning with replacement. These findings are not without contradictory data also being available in the literature. Basson (31) noted that although estrogen deficiency can impair sexual response, placing a patient on it may not improve sexual symptoms and may in fact exacerbate them; post-hysterectomy women can experience poor sexual functioning even on standard estrogen replacement regimens (32). There are also problems with the research designs of some of the investigations in this area. Walling et al. reviewed the literature on hormone replacement and sexual functioning and identified several design problems in the research: (a) There is often a lack of control for age and subjects are often not categorized by the number of years they have been postmenopausal. (b) Perimenopausal and postmenopausal women are often included in the same group. (c) Many studies that do not have a placebo control group (33).

B. Progestins and Progesterone

Certainly, the majority of women who are still prescribed exogenous estrogens in the perimenopause are prescribed a low-dose combination oral contraceptive preparation, so it is important to also describe important effects of synthetic progestins. Progestins influence important symptoms that women may experience in some phases of the perimenopause. Progestin use can reduce menorrhagia as a result of eventual endometrial secretory exhaustion, but may increase PMS symptoms of dysphoria, headaches, and water retention, due to decreased blood levels of progesterone (34). In terms of the painful uterine contractions that some peri/postmenopausal women can have during orgasm, progesterone as well as estrogen replacement are required to treat this condition (3). Natural micronized progesterone has not been shown to increase PMS and a brain mapping experiment showed changes in brain activity with natural progesterone that could exert positive effects on mood and cognitive changes associated with the perimenopause (34).

C. Androgens

Androgens also play a clear role in sexual arousal and functioning and a number of studies have explored the value of androgen supplementation for some women to increase and maintain sex drive and functioning. Testosterone replacement can positively affect libido, sexual arousal, and sexual fantasies and may be essential in restoring normal sexual functioning in ovariectomized or peri- or postmenopausal women. Pearce and Hawton reported that both estrogens and androgens have shown to have positive effects on libido, but the effect is especially clear for surgically menopausal women (35). Shifren et al. noted that women who were treated with 150 and 300 mcg of transdermally administered testosterone per day, although having an appreciable placebo response, had improvements in the frequency of sexual activity, sexual pleasure, and orgasm at the higher dose (36). In addition, positive well-being, depressed mood, and composite scores of the psychological general well-being index improved at the higher dose of transdermal testosterone. Basson also supports the notion that androgen supplementation may restore sexual responding and libido; suggests diagnosing testosterone deficiency based on a low level of free testosterone; and notes that avoiding alkylated testosterone lessens hepatic or lipid impairment (31). Other researchers have been skeptical about the role of decreased testosterone exerting a role on sexual functioning in the perimenopause, citing troublesome side effects of acne, hirsuitism, alopecia, bloating, and undesirable changes in lipids (37). Also, as the potentially harmful side effects of testosterone supplementation have not been adequately studied, some physicians are understandably cautious about prescribing exogenous testosterone. The use of tibolone has also been shown to significantly improve well-being, vasomotor symptoms, and vaginal dryness in natural postmenopausal women and, similar to estrogen replacement with progesterone, tibolone increases both sexual desire and the frequency of intercourse (38). As a counter argument, Burger et al. noted that the amount of bioavailable testosterone (measured by the free androgen index) is actually greater during perimenopause than prior to this phase of the life cycle, prompting these researchers to postulate that changes in sexual function during the perimenopause are not associated with a testosterone decline (39).

IV. PRIMARY CARE ASSESSMENT AND TREATMENT FOR PERIMENOPAUSAL PROBLEMS

A. History and Physical Examination Regarding Sexual Functioning

As sexual functioning is an important ingredient in the quality of life for many peri/postmenopausal women, clinicians should view the evaluation of sexual function as an essential part of comprehensive medical encounters. Although potentially anxiety-producing for both physicians and patients, a non-judgmental, matter-of-fact approach to obtaining a sexual history can be comfortable for most (40). Bachmann suggests that an abbreviated sexual history consisting of two questions can help the gynecologist, primary care physician, or other women's health provider identify women who may need help with sexual problems. She identifies these two questions: "Are you sexually active?" and "Are you having any sexual difficulties such as pain with intercourse, lack of sexual desire, or a decrease in vaginal lubrication with sexual arousal?" (25). Mazer et al. noted that a brief index of sexual functioning for women (BISF-W) is a questionnaire that can catalogue sexual difficulties in women and allow clinicians to identify potential areas of problems. Other researchers (15) have developed an index which can serve as an outcome measure to document the efficacy of a medical intervention when treating sexual dysfunction

Given the changes that can occur during the climacteric, the physician or other medical provider should examine the vulva and vagina for signs of atrophy. Notable among these are pale and friable tissues; vaginal inflammation as evidenced by erythema, petechia, bleeding, or increased vascularity; vulvar irritation; a change in the position of the external urethral meatus; and assessing vaginal pH in the proximal third. In addition, the clinician should look for signs of prolapse in major structures, including cystocele, rectocele, and uterine or urethral prolapse (37).

B. Education About Sexual Functioning and the Role of Counseling

Primary care physicians, obstetricians/gynecologists, psychotherapists, nurse practitioners, and other health professionals can employ essential elements of behavioral sex therapy techniques and tailor them to problems in the perimenopause. Education by discussion and by bibliotherapy using relevant materials is crucial. Reassurance about the normalcy of certain responses can be therapeutic for mid-life women. Brief primary care counseling can address changes in sexual interactions between couples, focusing on the need for longer and more intense foreplay techniques, adaptation to greater sensitivity to touch, the consistent use of effective vaginal lubricants, and realistic expectations regarding orgasmic phase responding. If more intensive treatment is required, referral to an appropriate health professional who specializes in behavioral sex therapy should result in successful outcomes for patients in a limited number of counseling sessions. Specific behavioral sex therapy approaches, such as altering physical alignment during coition, have been shown to improve sexual desire and orgasm (41).

C. Sexual Activity, Physical Activity, and Sexual Health

It is also important to note that regular sexual activity is one of the best behavioral strategies to maintain healthy sexual functioning. As Dr. Masters used to comment regarding male sexual functioning, "Use it or lose it." Pearce and Hawton note that, although both estrogens and androgens are beneficial in restoring a normal vaginal flora and lubrication during sexual activity, regular continued sexual activity is also able to serve as a prophylaxis against vaginal dryness. Li et al. found that women who were at least moderately physically active reported fewer symptoms during the perimenopause, including sexual symptoms, such as vaginal dryness, and lowered libido (42). They conclude that regular physical exercise might serve as an alternative to hormonal therapy for sexual symptoms management during the perimenopause. Other researchers have investigated the effect of physical exertion (which would activate the sympathetic nervous system) immediately prior to exposure to sexual stimuli and found that exercise increased two physiological measures of arousal in women, including vaginal blood volume (43). Although exercise did not affect perceived sexual desire in dysfunctional women, it clearly was shown to affect genital sexual responses.

D. Dysfunction in the Interpersonal Relationship

All primary care providers who evaluate and treat women with sexual concerns need to address other important areas. First, it is essential to underscore that a troubled sexual relationship may be a symptom of a troubled couple relationship. Clinicians need to be sensitive to issues of couple discord and assess whether relationship issues might be the cause of the woman's sexual complaints. In examining physical symptoms, emotional symptoms, and marital satisfaction, it was shown that there was a significant negative association between marital satisfaction and menopausal symptomatology (44). Other researchers noted that, in women with partners, sexual satisfaction, frequency of sexual activities, and orgasm were more highly associated with marital adjustment than with their menopausal phase (29). Excellent discussions of work on the interconnection of relationship issues and sexual functioning can be found in other sources (3–5) and will not be described in detail here. In summary, however, as well as being an expression of affection, intimacy, and couple bonding; sex can be used as an instrument of rejection, criticism, power, and control. For women, secondary anorgasmia has been shown to be related to relationship variables, whereas primary anorgasmia has not. Sexual problems and problems in couple dynamics occur in both heterosexual women and lesbians and all health providers should be able to discuss these problems and provide information to women, regardless of their affectional and sexual alliances. If relationship discord or disaffection is the primary problem, the woman should first be referred to a psychotherapist for couple counseling with her partner, not offered advice regarding the sexual problems. Providers also need to be alert to the possible presence of serious family issues such as infidelity and domestic violence. If these more complex issues are uncovered during discussion, the patient should be referred to a mental health professional who specializes in the management of these types of interpersonal dynamics. Physicians also need to counsel all women about issues of sexual health, being especially cognizant of the possibility of sexually transmitted diseases in situations where women or their partners have multiple sexual partners. STDs are not limited to the young, and mid-life women who are at risk need to be educated and provided with appropriate safety measures (45).

E. Domestic Violence

In reviewing the research on violence against women, Kosch and Dewar emphasized that intimate partner violence directed against women is highly prevalent, with 25% to 30% of all primary care patients and emergency department patients having experienced abuse within the last year (46). Over their lifetimes, 25% of women will sustain injuries connected to domestic violence, and of rape victims over 30 years of age, 50% have been sexually violated by their husbands or intimate partners. Domestic violence is more frequent in younger women, with one study documenting a 44% incidence in the last 12 months in primary care women patients under the age of 25 and an 11% incidence in those older than 25 (47). The frequency in perimenopausal women, then, is lower than in younger women, but a history of possible abuse should still be explored in this age group. Studies have shown that direct questions about abuse are highly sensitive and specific in its detection and that patients are comfortable with providers asking directly about abuse. Two questions with high sensitivity/specificity include the following high severity question: "Within the last year, have you been hit, slapped, kicked, or physically hurt by someone. If so, by who?" and the low severity question "Within the last year, have you been pushed, grabbed, or have you or someone you love been threatened?" (48). A "warm up" statement that normalizes abuse may make a person experience less discomfort discussing it with the provider: "I now ask all of my patients about safety issues, as I realize that discord in families often leads to physical conflict." A sensitive inquiry into any forced/coercive sexual activities is also warranted.

F. When a Male Partner Has Sexual Problems

If a clinician discovers that a woman's problem with sexual functioning is connected to a sexual dysfunction in a male partner, she/he can provide brief education and counseling about expected changes in aging males: (a) a greater need for consistent physical stimulation during sexual activities to obtain and maintain erections, (b) a longer latency between ejaculation and the ability to obtain another erection—an increased refractory period, (c) a possible diminution in ejaculatory volume and force, and (d) potential treatment options for male sexual dysfunction. In addition, maintaining a referral network of appropriate primary care providers, urologists, and psychotherapists who routinely treat male sexual dysfunctions is essential. It is important to note a current phenomenon that has been observed by health care providers, as they see mid-life couples in their practices. When men are prescribed any of the three phosphodiesterase type 5 inhibitors—sildenafil (Viagra), vardenafil (Levitra), or tadalafil (Cialis)—for erectile dysfunction, their spouses/partners may experience distress with the men's demands for intercourse of increased frequency or duration. In fact, the women partners may have been comfortable with a reduced frequency or a shorter duration coition, as their own perimenopausal changes created a situation that was best adapted to less frequent, brief intercourse. Physicians need to be cognizant of this phenomenon and realize that when they significantly improve the sexual functioning of a man by prescribing a medication to change erectile response, his spouse/partner may experience a deterioration of her ability to function. This may lead to serious relationship issues in a union that was previously satisfactory and stable. This situation underscores the benefit of family-oriented care wherein health care providers include both partners in discussions about the medical care of each.

G. Medical Conditions and Sexual Dysfunction

A wide variety of medical conditions and the treatment protocols used in managing these conditions can lead to sexual dysfunction. For instance, many physicians are familiar with the elevated rate of impotence in men who have been insulin-dependent diabetics for a number of years. Women diabetics may also have lowered libido and difficulties with the sexual response cycle, due to neurological, vascular, or endocrine changes. Coronary artery disease can affect blood flow to the vaginal vault and clitoris, which is necessary for female sexual responding, just as it can prevent erection in men (49). Pulmonary disease may prevent a woman from reaching orgasm due to an inability to maintain high levels of sexual tension when dyspnea occurs. Surgery, including hysterectomy, vaginal resection for vulvar cancer, and surgery for cervical cancer can also affect sexual functioning, at least temporarily close to the time of surgery. If pelvic surgery damages any of the nerve or vascular supply to the vagina or clitoris, it can create permanent problems in sexual functioning. However, studies have shown the effect of confounding variables in sexual impairment due to hysterectomy (50) or that hysterectomy may even be associated with an improvement in sexual function (51). In addition, a number of medical treatments, including chemotherapy and abdominal or pelvic radiation can affect libido and the ability of women to achieve orgasm, either through alterations in hormone levels (tamoxifen) or by creating vaginal atrophy (52).

Many types of commonly prescribed medications have been shown to be associated with an increased risk of sexual dysfunction in women, including antihistamines, antihypertensives, anticholinergics, anticonvulsants, narcotics, psychotropic medications (antipsychotics, antidepressants, and anxiolytics), and oral contraceptives (49). One of the most important areas of interface between medications and sexual dysfunctions involves selective serotonin re-uptake inhibitors (SSRIs), due to this category being the most frequently prescribed type of medication in the United States. Recent research has clearly demonstrated that a significant number of patients taking SSRIs have problematic sexual side effects. Labbate et al. reported that over 60% of both men and women had sexual side effects on sertraline (Zoloft), paroxetine (Paxil), and fluoxetine (Prozac), including decreases in sexual frequency, libido, lubrication, delayed orgasm, orgasms of poorer quality, or anorgasmia (53). Research has shown that a regimen of buproprion (Wellbutrin) can successfully decrease the sexual side effects of the SSRIs (54). Ashton and Rosen recommended a protocol in which the patient takes 75 to 150 mg of Wellbutrin one to two hour(s) prior to sexual activity. A second protocol involves titrating the patient up to a buproprion dose of 75 mg/day for at least two weeks. Nelson, Keck, and McElroy reported a 50% improvement in sexual functioning after one month on this regimen (55). The tricyclic antidepressant trazedone also has been demonstrated to resolve SSRI-induced lowered libido and anorgasmia (56). On the other hand, other reports and research document no benefit of adding antidepressants, including bupropion SR, over a number of weeks versus placebo in the ability of women to improve sexual functioning (57,58). Nurnberg et al. had good results with a small sample of women who were prescribed 50 mg of sildenafil (Viagra), taken one hour before sexual activity (59). In those women who were not assisted by 50 mg, a 100-mg dose proved effective. Ashton also reported that sildenafil was of benefit to women with paroxetine-induced sexual dysfunction (60).

In addition to the use of SSRIs for depression and anxiety, they are now being prescribed "off label" for peri- and menopausal symptoms. With all of the research focused on the risks of hormone replacement therapy, many physicians have been substituting a prescription for an SSRI rather than HRT to control vasomotor symptoms that occur in the perimenopause. Being aware of the high rate of sexual dysfunction associated with the SSRIs is important, as the benefit of improving hot flashes may be counterbalanced by an increased risk of anorgasmia.

H. Medical Treatments

In 2000, the FDA approved a device known as the EROS-CVD, which is a clitoral vacuum device, to assist women in the arousal phase of the sexual response cycle. It involves a suction cup and uses a battery to create suction to increase blood flow to the clitoris, which, in turn, leads to heightened sensory input from the clitoral body and elicits vaginal lubrication (61). Research on the use of a nasally administered apomorphine for the treatment of sexual dysfunction in women is currently in a phase II trial of safety. Apomorphine is thought to act as a dopamine agonist that stimulates the D1/D2 class of dopamine receptors in the midbrain. These receptors send efferent signals from brain down the spinal cord to increase vaginal/pelvic vasocongestion and increase libido; thus, raising both lubrication and tactile sensation. It is likely to be several years before adequate research trials on apomorphine are completed to apply for FDA approval in the United States, although this agent has already been approved for use in men with erectile dysfunction in Europe (62).

Given the connection between perimenopausal changes in hormonal status and increased difficulties in sexual functioning, women and their physicians are confronted with the advisability of using supplemental hormones to improve functioning. In its 2007 position statement, The North American Menopause Society noted that physicians should consider whether a patient's quality of life—including sexuality—was significantly altered when prescribing hormonal therapy for targeted goals. The Society further noted that treatment decisions should weigh potential benefits of estrogen and estrogen plus progestogen therapy with the risks of cardiovascular conditions and other diseases. It reported that research indicates a smaller risk of deep venous thrombosis (DVT) with transdermal estradiol as compared to oral estrogen, but not necessarily a difference in the slightly elevated breast cancer risk over untreated patients. Although oral ET/EPT agents are FDA-approved for treating moderate to severe vaginal atrophy and dyspareunia, the Society recommends using local topical products rather than systemic ones (63).

V. PATIENT EDUCATION SUMMARY

A. What is the Perimenopause?
A period of a woman's life when she experiences physiological changes related to the decrease of hormones produced by the ovaries: estrogen, progesterone, and testosterone.

B. When is the Perimenopause?
The period spans from the first symptoms of decreasing hormones to full ovarian failure. The average age of menopause is around 51 years of age, and most women experience symptoms for about five or six years prior to that. However, some women can begin the perimenopause much earlier, even during their 30s, and others do not reach menopause until they are beyond 55 years of age. Menopause is defined as 12 consecutive months without a menstrual period.

C. What Frequent Symptoms Do Women Experience Related to These Hormonal Changes?
Irregular menstrual cycles
Initially, a shortening of the cycle to around 21 days from around 28 days
Later, a lengthening of the cycles and skipped cycles
Periods may have heavier bleeding and some spotting before the period starts
Vasomotor symptoms (hot flashes or flushes) and night sweats
Insomnia
Fatigue
Changes in body appearance: Laxity or wrinkling of skin, relative decrease in muscle tone, a thickening of the waistline, loss of collagen tissue that changes breast shape.

Psychological Symptoms—Most women experience some distress with a change in body image and a sense of the beginning of aging. Many women handle these changes with aplomb. A caring and sensitive partner and a stable relationship can help minimize the distress of this life phase. About 25% of women experience depressive symptoms. Women with a history of anxiety symptoms or premenstrual symptoms may find that these worsen during this time period. The symptoms tend to resolve or return to baseline after menopause.

Cognitive Symptoms—Some, but not all, women report memory and concentration problems.

D. What Sexual Changes or Problems Do Women Experience in Perimenopause?

Sexual desire usually remains about the same

Reduced sexual activity

Reduced enjoyment in sexual activities

Increased sensitivity to touch—skin contact can be irritating

Reduced vaginal lubrication; increased dryness

Higher likelihood of dyspareunia—pain with vaginal penetration

More difficulty reaching high levels of sexual arousal

More difficulty obtaining orgasm

Orgasmic response is less intense

E. What Treatments Are Available to Help With the Sexual Changes of Perimenopause?

All women benefit from maintaining a regular aerobic exercise plan, those who exercise preserve sexual functioning compared to those who do not. Maintaining an active sex life also shows a benefit in sexual functioning over those who infrequently engage in sexual activities. For the major problem of vaginal dryness, the use of suppositories that simulate vaginal secretions and the liberal application of an effective lubricant during sexual activities are highly beneficial. Hormone therapies can significantly affect sexual functioning during the perimenopause. Many physicians prescribe low-dose oral contraceptives and this can help maintain vaginal health and reduce problematic menstrual cycles that occur during the perimenopause. Hormone-based creams prescribed by physicians can also be helpful to vaginal health and sexual functioning. Psychological counseling with a psychologist, psychiatrist, or other mental health professional specifically experienced in the treatment of sexual dysfunctions may be indicated. Behavioral sex therapy has been utilized and researched since the 1970s and has been shown to be highly effective. There is a vacuum device designed to increase blood flow to the genitalia that is FDA approved for patients with sexual arousal disorders, called EROS-CVD. A physician can also prescribe "off label" medications that can increase vaginal blood flow and lubrication; these medications may be ones approved for use in men with dysfunction.

F. A Friend Told Me that Her Physician Prescribed an SSRI for Hot Flashes? Should I Consider This?

Since the recent controversy about the benefits and risks of hormone replacement therapy, many physicians have been prescribing SSRIs for the vasomotor symptoms occurring in the perimenopause. One problem with the SSRIs is that many women experience anorgasmia on them and a number of women also experience lowered libido. These side effects can be managed by adding a second medication to assist with sexual functioning, such as another type of antidepressant.

REFERENCES

1. Peterson DD, Schmidt RM. Longitudinal and cross-sectional analysis of HEALTH WATCH data with a subset of perimenopausal women and matched controls. J Gerontol A Biol Sci Med Sci 1999; 54(4):B160–170.
2. Sulak PJ. The perimenopause: a critical time in a woman's life. Int J Fertil Menopausal Stud 1996; 41(2):85–89.
3. Masters WH, Johnson VE. Human Sexual Response. Boston: Little, Brown and Company, 1966.

4. Masters WH, Johnson VE. Human Sexual Inadequacy. Boston: Little, Brown and Company, 1970.
5. Kaplan HS. The New Sex Therapy: Active Treatment of Sexual Dysfunctions. New York: Brunner/Mazel Publications, 1974.
6. Barbach L. For Yourself: The Fulfillment of Female Sexuality. New York: Doubleday, 1976.
7. Moynihan R. The making of a disease: female sexual dysfunction. BMJ 2003; 326:45–47.
8. Kaschak E, Tiefer L (eds). A New View of Women's Sexual Problems. New York, NY: The Haworth Press; 2001.
9. Read S, King M, Watson J. Sexual dysfunction in primary medical care: prevalence, characteristics and detection by the general practitioner. J Public Health Med 1997; 19(4):387–391.
10. Basson R, Berman J, Burnett A et al. Report of the international consensus development conference on female sexual dysfunction: definitions and classifications. J Urol 2000; 163(3): 888–893.
11. Heiman JR. Sexual dysfunctions: Overview of prevalence, etiological factors and treatments. J Sex Res 2002; 39:73–78.
12. Heiman JR, LoPiccolo J, Palladini D. Becoming Orgasmic: A Sexual and Personal Growth Program for Women. Revised. New York: Fireside, 1988.
13. Binik YM, Pukall CF, Reissing ED et al. The sexual pain disorders: a desexualized approach. J Sex Marital Ther 2001; 27(2):113–116.
14. Bachmann GA. Sexual function in the perimenopause. Obstet Gynecol Clin North Am 1993; 20(2):379–389.
15. Berman JR, Berman LA, Werbin TJ et al. Clinical evaluation of female sexual function: effects of age and estrogen status on subjective and physiologic sexual responses. Int J Impot Res 1999; 11(Suppl 1):31–38.
16. Nachtigall LE. The symptoms of perimenopause. Clin Obstet Gynecol 1998; 41(4): 921–927.
17. LeBoeuf FJ, Carter SG. Discomforts of the perimenopause. J Obstet Gynecol Neonatal Nurs 1996; 25:173–180.
18. Pariser SF, Niedermier JA. Sex and the mature woman. J Womens Health 1998; 7(7): 849–859.
19. Lichtman R. Perimenopausal and postmenopausal hormone replacement therapy. Part 2. Hormonal regimens and complementary and alternative therapies. J Nurse Midwifery 1996; 41(3):195–210.
20. Koster A, Garde K. Sexual desire and menopausal development. A prospective study of Danish women born in 1936. Maturitas 1993; 16:49–60.
21. Avis NE, Stellato R, Crawford S et al. Is there an association between menopause status and sexual functioning? Menopause 2000; 7(5):297–309.
22. Hollingworth BA, Guillebaud J. Contraception in the perimenopause. Br J Hosp Med 1991; 45(4):213–215.
23. Koonin LM, Smith JC, Ramick M. Abortion surveillance—United States, 1991. Mor Mortal Wkly Rep CDC Surveill Summ 1995; 44(2):23–53.
24. Dennerstein L, Dudley E, Burger H. Are changes in sexual functioning during midlife due to aging or menopause? Fertil Steril 2001; 76(3):456–460.
25. Bachmann GA. Sexual issues at menopause. Ann NY Acad Sci 1990; 592:87–94.
26. Diokno AC, Brown MB, Herzog AR. Sexual function in the elderly. Arch Intern Med 1990; 150(1):197–200.
27. Sarrel PM. Psychosexual effects of menopause: role of androgens. Am J Obstet Gynecol 1999; 180(3 Pt 2):S319–S324.
28. Huerta R, Mena A, Malacara JM et al. Symptoms at the menopausal and premenopausal years: their relationship with insulin, glucose, cortisol, FSH, prolactin, obesity and attitudes towards sexuality. Psychoneuroendocrinology 1995; 20(8):851–864.
29. Hawton K, Gath D, Day A. Sexual function in a community sample of middle-aged women with partners: effects of age, marital, socioeconomic, psychiatric, gynecological, and menopausal factors. Arch Sex Behav 1994; 23:375–395.
30. Semmens JP, Wagner G. Estrogen deprivation and vaginal function in postmenopausal women. JAMA 1982; 248(4):445–448.

31. Basson R. Androgen replacement for women. Can Fam Physician 1999; 45:2100–2107.
32. Mazer NA, Leiblum SR, Rosen RC. The brief index of sexual functioning for women (BISF-W): a new scoring algorithm and comparison of normative and surgically menopausal populations. Menopause 2000; 7(5):350–363.
33. Walling M, Andersen BL, Johnson SR. Hormonal replacement therapy for postmenopausal women: a review of sexual outcomes and related gynecologic effects. Arch Sex Behav 1990; 19(2):119–137.
34. Martorano JT, Ahlgrimm M, Colbert T. Differentiating between natural progesterone and synthetic progestins: clinical implications for premenstrual syndrome and perimenopause management. Compr Ther 1998; 24(6–7):336–339.
35. Pearce MJ, Hawton K. Psychological and sexual aspects of the menopause and HRT. Baillieres Clin Obstet Gynaecol 1996; 10(3):385–399.
36. Shifren JL, Braunstein GD, Simon JA et al. Transdermal testosterone treatment in women with impaired sexual function after oophorectomy. N Engl J Med 2000; 343(10):682–688.
37. Leclair DM, Anandarajah G. Effects of estrogen deprivation: vasomotor symptoms, urogenital atrophy and psychobiologic effects. Clin Fam Prac 2002; 4(1):27–39.
38. Egarter C, Topcuoglu AM, Vogl S et al. Hormone replacement therapy with tibolone: effects on sexual functioning in postmenopausal women. Acta Obstet Gynecol Scand 2002; 81(7):649–653.
39. Burger HG, Dudley EC, Cui J. A prospective longitudinal study of serum testosterone, dhydroepiandrosterone sulfate, and sex hormone-binding globulin levels through the menopause transition. J Clin Endocrinol Metab 2000; 85:2832–2838.
40. Andrews WC. Approaches to taking a sexual history. J Womens Health Gend Based Med 2000; 9(Suppl1):S21–S24.
41. Pierce AP. The coital alignment technique (CAT): an overview of studies. J Sex Marital Ther 2000; 26(3):257–268.
42. Li S, Holm K, Gulanick M et al. Perimenopause and the quality of life. Clin Nurs Res 2000; 9(1):6–23.
43. Meston CM, Gorzalka BB. Differential effects of sympathetic activation on sexual arousal in sexually dysfunctional and functional women. J Abnorm Psychol 1996; 105(4):582–591.
44. Kurpius SER, Nicpon MF, Maresh SE. Mood, marriage, and menopause. J Couns Psychol 2001; 48(1):77–84.
45. Hatcher RA, Trussell J, Stewart F et al. Contraceptive Technology. New York: Ardent Media, Inc., 1998.
46. Kosch SG, Dewar MA. Domestic violence—2001. (Audiotape). Birmingham, Alabama: Educational Reviews, Inc., 2001.
47. Gin NE, Rucker L, Frayne S et al. Domestic violence prevalence of domestic violence among patients in three ambulatory care internal medicine clinics. J Gen Intern Med 1991; 6(4):317–322.
48. Feldhaus KM, Koziol-McLain J, Amsbury HL et al. Accuracy of 3 brief screening questions for detecting partner violence in the emergency department. JAMA 1997; 277(17):1357–1361.
49. Brassil DF, Keller M. Female sexual dysfunction: definition, causes, and treatment. Urologic Nursing 2002; 22(4):237–246.
50. Farrell SA, Kieser K. Sexuality after hysterectomy. Obstet Gynecol 2000; 95(6 Pt 2): 1045–1051.
51. Rhodes JC, Kjerulff KH, Langenberg PW et al. Hysterectomy and sexual functioning. JAMA 1999; 282(20):1934–1941.
52. Mortimer JE, Boucher L, Batay J et al. Effect of tamoxifen on sexual functioning in patients with breast cancer. J Clin Oncol 1999; 17(5):1488–1492.
53. Labbate LA, Grimes J, Hines A et al. Sexual dysfunction induced by serotonin reputake antidepressants. J Sex Marital Ther 1998; 24(1):3–12.
54. Ashton AK, Rosen RC. Bupropion as an antidote for serotonin reuptake inhibitor-induced sexual dysfunction. J Clin Psychiatry 1998; 59(3):112–115.
55. Nelson EB, Keck PE Jr, McElroy SL. Resolution of fluoxetine-induced sexual dysfunction with the 5-HT3 antagonist granisetron. J Clin Psychiatry 1997; 58(11):496–497.
56. Michael A, O'Donnell EA. Fluoxetine-induced sexual dysfunction reversed by trazodone. Can J Psychiatry 2000; 45(9):847–848.

57. Brill M. Antidepressants and sexual dysfunction. sexuality reproduction & menopause: a publication of the American Society for Reproductive Medicine 2004; 2(1):35–40.

58. Masard PS, Ashton AK, Gupta S, Frank B. Sustained-release bupropion for selective serotonin reuptake inhibitor-induced sexual dysfunction (a randomized, double-blind, placebo-controlled, parallel group study). Am J Psychiatry 2001; 58:805–807.

59. Nurnberg HG, Hensley PL, Lauriello J et al. Sildenafil for women patients with antidepressant-induced sexual dysfunction. Psychiatr Serv 1999; 50(8):1076–1078.

60. Ashton AK. Sildenafil treatment of paroxetine-induced anorgasmia in a woman. Am J Psychiatry 1999; 156(5):800.

61. Berman JR, Berman LA. For Women Only: A Revolutionary Guide to Overcoming Sexual Dysfunction and Reclaiming Your Sex Life. New York: Henry Holt and Company, 2001.

62. Health and Medicine Week. Agreement reached to develop and market nasally administered apomorphine. March 18, 2002, p. 5.

63. The North American Menopause Society. Estrogen and progestogen use in peri- and post-menopausal women: March 2007 position statement of The North American Menopause Society. Menopause: The Journal of The North American Menopause Society 2007; 14(2):168–182.

8

Urinary Incontinence in the Perimenopausal Patient

I. Keith Stone
Department of Obstetrics and Gynecology, University of Florida College of Medicine, Gainesville, Florida, U.S.A.

Joseph M. Novi
Department of Urogynecology and Reconstructive Pelvic Surgery, Riverside Methodist Hospital, Columbus, Ohio, U.S.A.

I. INTRODUCTION

Urinary incontinence is a common and underreported problem affecting women of all ages. It is defined by the International Continence Society as "the complaint of any involuntary leakage of urine that is objectively demonstrable and is a social and hygienic problem" (1). The annual direct cost of treating urinary incontinence in the United States in 2000 was estimated to be 19.5 billion dollars (2).

The prevalence of urinary incontinence ranges up to 54.4% depending on the definition used and the population studied, with a mean prevalence of 27.6% (3). Harrison and Memel (1994) published a questionnaire study of women aged 20 to 80. Of note, in that study the prevalence of urinary incontinence in women between the ages of 20 and 49 was found to be 47% (4). It is estimated that less than half of all women with urinary incontinence will bring this complaint to the attention of a medical practitioner (5). Table 1 lists the most common types of urinary incontinence in perimenopausal women.

II. RISK FACTORS FOR URINARY INCONTINENCE

Multiple risk factors have been found to be associated with urinary incontinence. These include age, parity, vaginal delivery, obesity, race, and lifestyle factors.

1. *Age:* Several studies have identified increasing age as a major risk factor in the development of urinary incontinence. A recent review of the literature showed that

Table 1 Most Common Types of Urinary
Incontinence in Perimenopausal Women

Stress Incontinence (SUI)
Urge Incontinence (UUI)
Mixed
Overflow
Fistula/Ectopic Ureter
Urethral Diverticulum

the median prevalence of any urinary incontinence peaks at two age groups, one in the fifth decade, and the second in the eighth decade. The prevalence of significant urinary incontinence increases from the second to the eighth decades (3).

2. *Pregnancy-related factors:* Almost 33% of women report stress urinary incontinence during pregnancy and most tend to be new onset. It has been shown that the risk of having urinary incontinence five years postpartum was increased in women who developed stress urinary incontinence during the first pregnancy and in women who developed stress incontinence during the first six weeks postpartum (6). Multiparity and vaginal delivery have also been shown to be independently associated with an increased risk of having urinary incontinence later on in life (3,6). In addition, forceps-assisted vaginal delivery has also been associated with a higher risk of urinary incontinence (7). Data regarding size of baby, fetal head, etc., is controversial (6).

3. *Obesity:* Increased body mass index (BMI) has been established as an independent risk factor for the development of urinary incontinence. It has been shown that with each unit increase in BMI, there is a 5% increase in the odds of having urinary leakage (8).

4. *Race:* Several studies have investigated the relationship between ethnicity, and urinary incontinence. After adjusting for known risk factors such as age, parity, and BMI, the data demonstrated that Caucasian race is a significant risk factor for stress urinary incontinence (3,6,9). In one study, African-American race was a significant predictor of urge incontinence (OR 2.6, 95% CI 1.45–4.80) (9).

5. *Diet:* Dietary factors that have been studied include carbonated beverages, caffeine, and alcohol intake. In a large longitudinal study, daily or more frequent intake of carbonated beverages was found to be a risk factor for stress urinary incontinence (OR 1.62, 95% CI 1.18–2.22) (10). Interestingly, in the same study, daily bread intake was found to be associated with a reduced risk of stress urinary incontinence (OR 0.76, 95% CI 0.61–0.96). High caffeine intake has also been associated with a higher risk of urge urinary incontinence (OR 2.4, 95% CI 1.1–6.5) (6,11,12). However, no statistically significant correlation between urinary incontinence and alcohol intake has been noted (3). One study has shown that eating disorders, such as anorexia nervosa, was associated with increased risk of all urinary symptoms including urgency, frequency, nocturia, stress, and urge urinary incontinence (13). This observation was supported in a study by Bo et al. (2001) (14). These authors reported an increased prevalence of stress urinary incontinence in athletes who had eating disorders (P = 0.03).

6. *Smoking:* Smoking has been shown to be a risk factor for both stress and urge urinary incontinence. It has been shown that women with overactive bladder were more likely to be current smokers than controls (11). Women smokers have also been reported to have a 2.5-fold increased risk of developing stress urinary incontinence (14) despite their stronger urethral sphincter and lower risk profile than nonsmokers (younger age and less hypoestrogenic) (15).

7.   *Exercise:* It is well known that urinary incontinence during physical activities is a common complaint; however, it is not clear whether exercise is a causative factor in the development of urinary incontinence (16). Ultra-high impact forms of exercise, such as parachute jumping, have been shown to increase the risk of urinary incontinence, presumably through damage to the pelvic floor supports (17).

A. Types of Urinary Incontinence in Perimenopausal Women

There are several types of incontinence common in women in the perimenopause. Most of these women with urinary incontinence will have one of the following types: stress urinary incontinence (SUI), overactive bladder (OAB), mixed incontinence, overflow incontinence, ectopic ureter/urinary fistula. Less commonly, incontinence may result from transient causes, which can be remembered by the mnemonic DIAPPERS (Table 2), developed by Resnick in 1990 (18). Addressing the underlying condition will often result in significant improvement of the incontinence.

B. Stress Urinary Incontinence (SUI)

The primary etiology for urinary incontinence in the perimenopausal woman is SUI, whether alone or in combination with urge incontinence (mixed incontinence) (9). The International Continence Society defines SUI as the involuntary loss of urine when, in the absence of a detrusor contraction, the intravesical pressure exceeds the intraurethral pressure (1). The main cause of SUI is loss of support of the bladder neck and urethra. Normally, these structures lie upon a firm "platform" of endopelvic fascia and anterior vaginal wall. Rises in intra-abdominal pressure result in pressure transmission to the anterior surface of the proximal urethra, which becomes compressed against this "platform," effectively sealing the urethra and preventing urine loss. Absent the normal supporting structures, intra-abdominal pressure is transmitted to the bladder and less effectively to the proximal urethra. This loss of support can be measured by use of the Q-tip test (Fig. 1) (19).

In patients with a well-functioning urethral sphincter, it is rare that the abdominal pressure would rise high enough to push urine through the urethra. However, if the external urethral sphincter is unable to maintain urethral closure when confronted with a rise in bladder pressure, urine loss will result. The intravesical pressure needed to overcome the urethral closure mechanism is called the valsalva leak point pressure (VLPP). This is measured during multichannel urodynamics using rectal and intravesical transducers. Normally the urethra can withstand pressures in the bladder of well over 100 cm of water without urine

Table 2 Causes of Transient Incontinence

Dementia
Infection
Atrophic vaginitis
Psychoses
Pharmaceuticals
Excess intake/excess output
Restricted mobility
Stool impaction

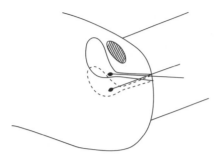

Figure 1 Q-tip test.

loss (20). However, in patients with altered urethral closure pressures, known as intrinsic sphincter deficiency, the VLPP may measure less than 60 cm of water (21).

C. Urge Urinary Incontinence (UUI)

Neurologic diseases (multiple sclerosis, cerebrovascular accidents, Parkinson's disease, Alzheimer's disease), foreign bodies (stones, suture material), previous anti-incontinence surgery, and urinary tract infections can all cause UUI. However, the most common cause is idiopathic overactive bladder (OAB). The hallmark of this syndrome is uninhibited detrusor (bladder muscle) contractions, typically at lower than normal bladder volumes. The diagnosis is best made on history and evaluation of a voiding diary, as urodynamic testing has been shown to be unreliable in demonstrating this condition (22).

Other important causes of UUI, including pharmacologic and nonpharmacologic agents, are frequently associated with heightened bladder activity and a sense of urgency. Any medication that affects the autonomic nervous system will impact the lower urinary tract. A partial list includes antihypertensives, antidepressants, sedative/hypnotics, decongestants, antihistamines, and caffeine. Cholinergic agents, such as metoclopromide used to stimulate bowel function, may also stimulate the bladder resulting in incontinence.

D. Mixed Incontinence

As noted above, a combination of SUI and UUI results in mixed incontinence. Women in this category experience urine loss associated with a rise in intra-abdominal pressure and uninhibited detrusor contractions. This group of patients will often present the greatest therapeutic challenge.

E. Overflow Incontinence

The most common type of urinary incontinence in men is overflow incontinence caused by bladder outlet obstruction from an enlarged prostate gland. True bladder outlet obstruction in women is rare, and most often a result of prior anti-incontinence surgery (23). However, bladder outlet obstruction in women can be a consequence of severe pelvic organ prolaps with resultant urethral "kinking," benign and malignant pelvic neoplasms, retroversion and incarceration of a gravid uterus, and fecal impaction. Overflow incontinence from bladder atony may be secondary to neurologic disease, medication use (anticholinergic agents, alpha- and beta-adrenergic agonists, calcium channel blockers), endocrine disease (diabetes mellitus, hypothyroidism), and decreased compliance (radiation fibrosis, interstitial cystitis). An important additional cause is detrusor-sphincter dyssynergia, usually of neurogenic origin, as seen in multiple sclerosis. The symptoms of overflow incontinence may manifest as SUI, UUI, or mixed UI, and the diagnosis is dependent upon the measurement of the postvoid residual volume.

F. Urinary Tract Fistulas, Ectopic Ureter, Urethral Diverticulum

The most common cause of urinary tract fistula in the industrialized world is prior pelvic surgery, particularly hysterectomy (24). Lower urinary tract (LUT) injuries are estimated to occur in upwards of 1% of all hysterectomies (25). With over 600,000 women undergoing this procedure annually in the United States, approximately 6000 are complicated by LUT injury. Unfortunately, the majority of these injuries occur during surgery for benign indications and most are unrecognized at the time of the initial surgery (26). Urinary loss occurring in the postoperative period should be considered as a possible fistula until proven otherwise (27).

In underdeveloped countries, limited access to trained medical practitioners often results in protracted childbirth. This may lead to injuries from prolonged compression of the lower urinary tract by an impacted fetal presenting part. These childbirth events can cause extensive tissue necrosis and account for the vast majority of urinary tract fistulas in these populations (28).

Less common causes of urinary incontinence in the perimenopausal age group involve malformations of the genitourinary tract. The most common abnormalities give rise to ectopic ureters. These ureteric openings can be found anywhere along the lower genital tract, from the vagina to the urethra. Most congenital malformations are diagnosed in younger age groups. Constant leakage in the absence of prior surgery should prompt an investigation for GU malformations.

Urethral diverticula are thought to occur from an obstruction of a paraurethral gland. Common symptoms include recurrent UTI, dyspareunia, urinary incontinence, dysuria, and postvoid dribbling, although some are asymptomatic. Most diverticula form along the posterior wall of the urethra and can be palpated during vaginal exam.

G. Evaluation of Urinary Incontinence

1. History

A thorough history is an integral part of the initial evaluation of the incontinent woman. It is helpful in identifying transient (reversible) causes of incontinence, and may help direct the subsequent work-up. Unfortunately, the patient history is notoriously poor at differentiating the type of incontinence. The history should be used to evaluate the impact of UI on the patient's quality of life, the patient's assessment of severity, previous testing and intervention, and the patient's expectations.

Table 3 lists questions that should be asked when evaluating urinary incontinence. Standardized questionnaires may also be helpful. Many practitioners find that having the patient fill out a 1- to 3-day voiding diary prior to the initial visit saves considerable time. The voiding diary (Fig. 2) records the amount of fluid intake, amount of urine per each voiding episode, frequency of voids, presence or absence of urgency, incontinence episodes, and events that precipitate urinary leakage. The improved accuracy of a voiding diary compared with the patient's recollection of her bladder habits has been documented (29). A fluid intake of greater than four liters per day should prompt an evaluation for diabetes insipidus.

Table 3 Recommended Questions

Do you lose urine with coughing, sneezing, laughing, etc?
Do you get up at night to empty your bladder? If so, how many times?
How often do you void during the day (or how many times do you void during the day)?
Do you have a sense of urgency that makes you need to hurry to the bathroom?
Do you ever lose urine on the way to the bathroom when you have urgency?
Do you lose urine without knowing it?
Do you lose urine in your sleep?
Do you lose urine during sexual intercourse or orgasm?
Do you lose urine when you stand up after voiding?
Have you had bladder or kidney infections?
Do you have pain before, during, or after you urinate?
Do you have difficulty starting your urine stream?

It is important to question the patient about certain medical conditions as they may preclude the use of anticholinergic medications. These conditions include, but are not limited to, closed-angle glaucoma, cardiac dysrhythmias, and postural hypotension.

2. Physical Examination

The physical examination of the incontinent woman should consist of a general examination with a focus on the female pelvic floor. The general examination includes a complete basic evaluation, neurologic exam, gait, and general strength and mobility. The routine gynecologic examination is augmented with attention to the pelvic floor.

3. Pelvic Exam

Assessment of pelvic organ prolapse should be documented using the Baden-Walker Halfway System (30) or the Pelvic Organ Prolapse-Quantification (POP-Q) system (31). Measurement of bladder neck hypermobility can be accomplished by placing a lubricated

Time	Amount Voided	Fluid Intake (amount)	Leakage (small, large)	Activity during leakage (urge, cough, sneeze, etc.)

Figure 2 Voiding diary.

Q-tip into the urethra (Fig. 1). A goniometer can then be used to measure the angle of deflection of the Q-tip relative to the floor. The starting angle is subtracted from the angle achieved at greatest valsalva to arrive at the deflection. A starting angle of greater than 40° or a change in deflection of greater than 20° implies hypermobility but is not diagnostic. The Q-tip test has been shown to have a sensitivity of only 25%, a specificity of 78%, and positive predictive value of 67% (19).

After examination in the supine position, the patient should be asked to stand and the bimanual exam repeated. Any prolapse will likely be exacerbated by this change of position.

4. Postvoid Residual Assessment

Measurement of residual urine volume immediately after voiding is the most accurate method to rule out overflow incontinence (23). A postvoid residual (PVR) volume less than 50 cc is generally considered normal, and greater than 200 cc abnormal (32). However, a significant proportion of patients will have a PVR somewhere between these extremes and clinical correlation is necessary. Any abnormal value should be rechecked at a different sitting to eliminate spurious results. Confirmed abnormal values require investigation of voiding function and bladder compliance via cystometrics.

5. Laboratory Studies

Several authors advocate the collection of a urine specimen for urinalysis with culture and sensitivity in all patients with urinary incontinence (23,33). While it is important to exclude infection as a cause of urinary incontinence, a less costly method of evaluating infection involves a urine dipstick test. The dipstick urinalysis has a negative predictive value of 97% to 99% for detecting bacteriuria, and a negative test reliably rules out infection, obviating the need for culture. However, the sensitivity of this test is considerably lower, and has a positive predictive value of 50% to 60% (34). In the presence of a positive dipstick test, a urine culture and sensitivity should be obtained.

Other laboratory tests may include serum glucose, BUN, creatinine, serum and urine osmolality, and electrolytes, depending upon the clinical scenario.

6. Simple Urodynamics

Simple urodynamics (Fig. 3), also known as "eyeball" urodynamics, are useful in screening patients for further complex evaluation. This test assesses bladder capacity, sensation, uninhibited detrusor contractions, and postvoid residual. It has limited usefulness in determining the precise cause of urinary incontinence, but may yield useful information about overactive bladder. A catheter is placed into the bladder and attached to a 100 cc syringe chamber. Sterile water in 60-cc aliquots is introduced into the bladder via the chamber. The meniscus is observed for rises occurring coincident with a sense of urgency and suggesting a detrusor contraction. When maximum capacity is reached, the catheter is removed. The patient is then asked to perform valsalva maneuvers in both the supine and standing positions and the urethral meatus is observed for urinary leakage.

7. Complex Urodynamics

The advanced evaluation of the incontinent woman involves several specialized tests under the general heading of complex urodynamics. These include uroflowmetry, subtracted cystometry, leak-point pressure, and videourodynamics. Table 4 lists the indications for

Table 4 Indications for Advanced Testing

Uncertain diagnosis
Failure to respond to adequate trial of therapy
Considering surgical intervention
Recurrent urinary loss after previous anti-incontinence surgery
Bladder pain syndromes
Neurologic disease
Abnormal postvoid residual volume
Fistula or diverticulum
Hematuria without infection
Prior pelvic radiation
Prior radical pelvic surgery

these tests. While not every patient needs this type of work-up, any patient in whom surgical therapy is planned should undergo this level of testing.

8. Uroflowmetry

This test evaluates the detrusor function as a measure of urine flow. The patient voids into a sensing device, and the maximum flow rate, total voiding time, and volume are measured. Evaluation of detrusor function is important in counseling patients regarding surgical outcomes. Patients with altered detrusor function are at higher risk of voiding dysfunction and urinary retention requiring intermittent self-catheterization after anti-incontinence surgery.

9. Subtracted Cystometry

Microtip pressure transducer catheters placed into the bladder lumen measure the intravesical pressure (a combination of both intra-abdominal pressure and detrusor pressure). The addition of a transducer in the rectum or vagina to measure abdominal pressure

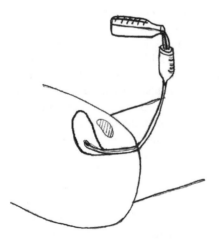

Figure 3 Eyeball urodynamics.

allows for an accurate estimate of true detrusor pressure by subtracting the abdominal pressure from intravesical pressure. This enhances the evaluation of uninhibited detrusor contractions (OAB) that may present as SUI.

10. Leak-point Pressure

The abdominal pressure (measured via rectal or vaginal transducer catheter) necessary to overcome the urethral sphincter and cause urinary leakage is the valsalva leak point pressure (VLPP). The VLPP is often helpful in choosing the correct procedure when surgical intervention for SUI is planned. Certain procedures for correction of bladder neck hypermobility, such as the Burch Retropubic Urethropexy, are thought to have diminished efficacy in the setting of intrinsic sphincter deficiency (35).

11. Videourodynamics

The addition of fluoroscopy to subtracted cystometry allows for the real-time evaluation of the bladder neck and pelvic organ anatomy at the time of assessment of detrusor function. This test is particularly helpful when physical findings and cystometry do not correlate with symptomatology.

12. Cystoscopy

All patients with irritative voiding symptoms (urgency, frequency, bladder pain), hematuria, and recurrent urinary incontinence should undergo cystoscopic evaluation of the lower urinary tract. Stones, polyps, mucosal abnormalities (including cancerous lesions), and retained suture material can be readily visualized. This test may be performed in an office setting. However, if a diagnosis of interstitial cystitis is suspected, cystoscopy with hydrodistention should be performed utilizing general anesthesia.

III. TREATMENT OF STRESS URINARY INCONTINENCE

A. Nonsurgical Therapies

Patients with urethral hypermobility and stress urinary incontinence may benefit from the insertion of a tampon into the vagina causing elevation of the bladder neck. Nygaard, in 1995, demonstrated a statistically significant reduction in urine loss during exercise associated with this "low-tech" approach (36). Additionally, a variety of pessaries exist that compress the urethra and elevate the bladder neck. Improvement rates of stress incontinence in the 30% to 70% range have been reported, though long-term use of these devices is uncommon (37).

Behavioral modification may certainly provide substantial improvement in the incontinent patient and avoid surgical intervention. Bladder retraining, timed voiding, pelvic muscle exercises, and electrical stimulation are all interventions that require dedication on the part of the patient and expertise on the part of the health care provider. This expertise may best be optimized when a close alliance exists with a physical therapist specializing in neuromuscular dysfunction of the pelvic floor.

1. Pelvic Floor Muscle Exercises (Kegel Exercises)

Several studies have demonstrated the efficacy of pelvic floor muscle exercises (38,39). When done properly, up to 70% of women have a significant improvement in their incontinence, with more than 30% reporting complete cure (39). Patients should be instructed to perform three sets of 10 exercises a day. Unfortunately, the benefit of these exercises is lost when the regimen is discontinued. The addition of biofeedback, a specialized teaching method utilized by physical therapists, may further improve success rates (40). Other options include weighted vaginal cones and functional electrical stimulation.

2. Hormonal Therapy

Estrogen therapy, both topical and oral preparations, has long been used to treat atrophic changes of the lower genital tract after menopause. Earlier studies reported improvement in SUI and UUI in women treated with hormonal medications (41). However, more recent studies suggest that hormone use after menopause did not improve subjective or objective outcomes of urinary incontinence (42) and may actually increase the risk for incontinence (43). In 1989, Bhatia et al. demonstrated an improvement in urethral closure pressures in women treated with estrogen vaginal cream, though incontinence rates before and after treatment were not statistically different (44). At present, the use of these medications for the treatment or prevention of urinary incontinence remains controversial.

B. Surgical Therapies

1. Retropubic Urethropexy

The mainstay of surgical treatment for SUI is the Burch retropubic urethropexy. Several long-term studies have documented 80% to 90% 5- and 10-year success rates (45,46). An abdominal incision (usually the transverse Pfannenstiel or the Cherney) is used to gain access to the retropubic region (space of Retzius). The urethrovesical junction is identified by locating the inflated intravesical Foley catheter balloon. With the operating surgeon's left hand in the vagina serving as a guide, the right hand is used to place the suspensory stitch(es) into the tissue plane 1 cm lateral to the urethra and 1 cm inferior to the bladder. This is accomplished on either side of the urethra and the suspensory stitches are secured to Cooper's ligament (the Burch procedure) or the periosteum of the symphysis pubis (the Marshall-Marchetti-Krantz procedure). The sutures are then tied loosely, providing support to the bladder neck without overcorrection (Fig. 4).

The retropubic urethropexy may be accomplished via laparoscopy, avoiding the transverse abdominal incision and using trocar inserted portals to accomplish needle/suture placement and urethral elevation. Laparoscopic retropubic urethropexy in the hands of accomplished surgeons has been reported to have similar initial success rates when compared with the open laparotomy approach (47).

2. Midurethral "Tension-Free" Sling

In the mid-1990s, Ulmsten and Petros in Sweden introduced the synthetic, tension-free, midurethral sling for the treatment of stress urinary incontinence (48). The procedure was first performed in the United States in the late 1990s, and has undergone an explosion of interest. Several similar products are now available with the same basic surgical precept: placement of the sling material in the midurethral region without tension. Success rates have been reported in the 80% to 90% range, with most procedures being done on an

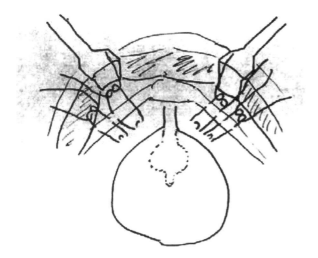

Figure 4 Burch retropubic urethropexy.

outpatient basis (49,50). Significant complications, such as bowel perforation and large vessel perforation, have been reported, but remain relatively rare (51).

With the patient in the lithotomy position, an incision is made through the vaginal mucosa overlying the urethra. The mucosa and muscularis layers are dissected away from the urethra and pubocervical fascia. Two 0.5-cm incisions are created through the abdominal skin at the upper margin of the pubic bone, 1 to 2 cm lateral to the midline. The bladder is drained and the sling introducer is placed against the inferior pubic ramus. The introducer is guided along the posterior surface of the pubic bone through the retropubic space, perforates the rectus fascia, and exits through the suprapubic skin incision on the ipsilateral side (Fig. 5). The procedure is repeated on the opposite side. Cystoscopy is imperative prior to advancing the sling material. If a bladder perforation is seen, the introducer is removed. It is reinserted after the bladder has again been drained. Prolonged catheter drainage of the bladder is not necessary after this type of perforation. After bladder injury has been excluded, the sling material is advanced and adjusted such that it lays in the midurethral region without tension. Care is taken not to elevate the urethra with the sling. Up to 70% of patients can be discharged without a catheter after an appropriate assessment of voiding function is done in the immediate postoperative period (50).

Approximately 1% to 5% of women undergoing midurethral sling placement will have significant voiding dysfunction consistent with obstruction (51,52). These cases are best managed by incising the sling in the midportion under the urethra. Small case series have reported that despite incision of the sling in this scenario, up to 80% of these women remain continent (53).

In an effort to decrease the occurrence of bladder injury, the transobturator approach has recently been employed. The basic principle of tension-free midurethral placement applies, but the needles are placed through the obturator foramen bilaterally instead of the retropubic space. Early experience is encouraging, with short-term success rates comparable to those seen with the traditional tension-free sling and the Burch procedure (54).

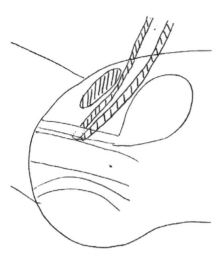

Figure 5 Tension-free midurethral sling.

The mechanism of action of the midurethral sling is controversial, with some investigators arguing that it is obstructive in nature while others feel it provides a static backboard for urethral compression. Recent studies in patients without urethral hypermobility have documented lower success rates (55).

3. Pubovaginal Sling

Patients with markedly reduced valsalva leak point pressures (less than 60 cm of water) may warrant placement of a pubovaginal sling to elevate the bladder neck. This traditional sling was first described by Von Giordano in 1907 (56), and popularized in the 1970s by McGuire (57). It is the procedure of choice for some practitioners and is the recommended treatment of recurrent SUI following anti-incontinence surgery. Multiple materials have been used and continue to be numerous: cadaveric fascia, tensor fascia lata (harvested from the patient just prior to the performance of the sling), anterior abdominal wall fascia, and Mersilene. Success rates are similar to those reported for retropubic procedures (58,59) and remain excellent even in women without urethral hypermobility (60). The pubovaginal sling requires a larger abdominal incision than the midurethral sling and suturing of the sling material to the rectus fascia.

4. Urethral Bulking Agents

Patients with low valsalva leak point pressures (less than 60 cm of water) and limited urethral mobility (nonmobile, "drainpipe" urethra) may benefit from trans-urethral or peri-urethral collagen injections. Collagen is injected under cystoscopic observation at the level of the proximal urethra to effect diminished lumen diameter and accomplish continence. The procedure may be performed in an office (cystoscopic suite) setting with minimal sedation and local anesthesia. Long-term results have been disappointing, with most patients requiring repeated injections (61). The maximum expected benefit appears to be limited to 18 to 24 months. Nonabsorbable materials have been used, but success rates are similar to collagen.

IV. TREATMENT OF URINARY URGE INCONTINENCE

A. Nonsurgical Therapies

1. Bladder Training (Timed Voids)

Bladder training includes both patient education and adherence to a voiding schedule. After completion of a voiding diary, the patient is asked to void during the day at a proscribed interval. If she senses urgency prior to the allotted time, she is instructed in several techniques, including pelvic floor exercises and relaxation drills, to inhibit urgency and postpone voiding. A trained physiotherapist with experience in pelvic floor disorders may be of particular assistance in this scenario. When the patient is able to void at the proscribed interval without experiencing urgency and/or incontinence, the interval is lengthened by 15 to 30 minutes. Fantl et al. (62) reported a 50% reduction in incontinence episodes in 75% of women using this intervention.

2. Dietary Modification

Limiting fluid intake may be helpful in women who consume excessive amounts of liquids. Eliminating or reducing intake of caffeine and carbonated beverages should be encouraged.

3. Pharmacologic Therapies

Anticholinergic medications are the mainstay of medical therapy for UUI/OAB. These compounds are relatively safe, effective, and have few contraindications (untreated narrow-angle glaucoma, cardiac arrhthymias). Common side effects include dry mouth, dry eyes, constipation, and somnolence. Table 5 includes dosages of medications used to treat UUI/OAB.

4. Oxybutynin Chloride

Oxybutynin was the first medication to undergo placebo-controlled trials for the treatment of UUI/OAB. It is available in a short-acting preparation, an extended release preparation, and a transdermal patch. All of these preparations have been shown to improve incontinence rates (63,64), though the short-acting form is associated with greater anticholinergic side effects (65).

Table 5 Medications Used in the Treatment of UUI/OAB

Generic name	Trade name	Dosage
Oxybutynin chloride (immediate release)	Ditropan IR	2.5–5 mg TID–QID
Oxybutynin chloride (extended release)	Ditropan XL	5–15 mg QID
Oxybutynin chloride (transdermal)	Oxytrol	3.9 mg/d patch applied twice weekly
Tolterodine tartrate (immediate release)	Detrol	1–2 mg BID
Tolterodine tartrate (extended release)	Detrol LA	2–4 mg QID
Trospium chloride (immediate release)	Sanctura	20 mg BID
Trospium chloride (extended release)	Sanctura XR	60 mg QID
Darifenacin	Enablex	7.5–15 mg QID
Solifenacin	Vesicare	5–10 mg QID
Hyoscyamine sulphate	Levsin, Levsinex	0.125 mg QID, 0.375 mg BID
Imipramine hydrochloride	Tofranil	10–50 mg BID

5. Tolterodine Tartrate

Tolterodine is available in an immediate release and extended release form. Both have been shown to significantly reduce urgency, frequency, and number of incontinence episodes. Trials comparing tolterodine to oxybutynin demonstrate equal efficacy between these medications (65,66), and some report decreased side effects with tolterodine (67,68).

6. Newer Anti-Muscarinic Medications

Three new medications are now available for the treatment of OAB, trospium chloride, solifenacin, and darifenicin. Each has placebo-controlled trials demonstrating its efficacy (69,70,71). Trospium, a quaternary amine, the only OAB medication that is metabolized by the renal system, is available in once daily and twice daily preparations. Darifenacin, given once daily, has the greatest affinity of all OAB medication for the M_3 receptor, theoretically reducing its potential for unwanted side effects. Solifenacin is available in 5 mg and 10 mg once daily dosages, allowing for flexible dosing.

7. Tricyclic Antidepressants

These medications have several distinct effects on the lower urinary tract. They have anticholinergic effects resulting in reduced urgency and frequency, but also increase urethral tone through their alpha-adrenergic properties. These medications can cause drowsiness, and may be helpful in treating women with significant nocturia. Use of tricyclic antidepressants in older women has been associated with orthostatic hypotension.

B. Surgical Therapy

1. Sacral Neuromodulation

Neuromodulation has been tried in several different forms, from anogenital electrical stimulation (72) and transcutaneous nerve stimulation to percutaneous posterior tibial nerve stimulation (73) and magnetic stimulation (74). All have been shown to be effective in treating UUI/OAB. However, the most effective neuromodulation is an implantable unit with stimulating electrodes placed in the S_3 foramen. Medtronic (Minneapolis, Minnesota) introduced InterStim therapy in 1997 and it is now being used to treat UUI/OAB, urinary retention, and lower urinary pain syndromes such as interstitial cystitis. Several authors have reported success rates of 50% to 75% using InterStim (75,76).

The appropriate candidate for sacral neuromodulation should undergo the complete urogynecologic evaluation and have tried conservative therapies without success. The implantation involves a two-step procedure. Initially, a test stimulator is placed and connected to a temporary stimulator. If the patient reports at least a 50% reduction in symptoms during a three- to five-day test period, the stimulator is then permanently implanted in the subcutaneous fat overlying the buttock. Changes in the frequency of stimulation can then be made using an external telemetry unit as necessary.

V. TREATMENT OF OTHER TYPES OF URINARY INCONTINENCE

A. Overflow Incontinence

Therapy for overflow incontinence is directed at the underlying cause. If obstruction is present due to severe prolapse, a pessary or surgical intervention should be considered.

If the patient has undergone a prior anti-incontinence procedure, urethrolysis or revision of the sling is warranted.

Overflow incontinence secondary to poor detrusor contractility may be treated with bethanechol, 25 to 100 mg four times daily. Bethanechol is a cholinergic agent that stimulates smooth muscle contractions. The side effects include flushing, nausea, vomiting, diarrhea, bronchospasm, headache, and visual changes which limits its usefulness. Published reports of the use of bethanechol in this setting have shown variable results (77). A regimen of intermittent self-catheterization of the bladder or an indwelling bladder catheter may be required.

B. Mixed Incontinence

The initial treatments of patients with SUI and UUI/OAB are typically directed at the predominating symptoms. Nonsurgical therapies that are effective in controlling both forms of incontinence should be tried first (pelvic floor exercises, biofeedback, bladder retraining, dietary modification). Published reports of the use of surgical interventions for SUI have also shown some improvement in UUI/OAB (78,79).

C. Ectopic Ureter/Genitourinary Fistula/Urethral Diverticulum

The primary treatment of urinary incontinence secondary to ectopic ureter, genitourinary fistulas, and urethral diverticula remains surgical. Occasionally, if a fistula is recognized early, prolonged (14 to 21 days) catheter drainage may result in spontaneous closure of the fistula (80,81).

D. Recommendations for Subspecialty Referral

Referral to a subspecialist (Urogynecologist or Urologist) should be considered for complex scenarios requiring advanced testing and interventions. These include: uncertain diagnosis, failure of initial therapy, recurrent UTI, hematuria, prior anti-incontinence procedure, suspected fistula or ectopic ureter, prior radical pelvic surgery, and prior pelvic radiation.

VI. SUMMARY

Urinary incontinence in the perimenopausal woman is a common and underreported condition. It does not have to be regarded as an inevitable part of aging. Effective treatments exist, and a substantial number of women will respond to noninvasive therapy. Questioning patients about incontinence and arriving at an accurate diagnosis are important steps in helping improve the quality of life of these women.

CASE STUDY 1

Profile: 67-year-old white female P3003

Chief Complaint: Urinary incontinence

History of Present Illness: The patient notes urinary incontinence for 10 years, with loss in small and large amounts several times a day. Leakage occurs with increased abdominal pressure, lifting, jarring motion, and upon hearing running water. She changes her pad and/or clothing once or twice a day. She has a prior sense of urgency. There is nocturia twice nightly. There are feelings of incomplete emptying and dribbling after urination.

<u>Prior Surgical History:</u> Abdominal hysterectomy and MMK urethropexy

<u>Past Medical History:</u> Gastric-esophageal reflux; hypertension

<u>Medications:</u> Synthroid®, Premarin®, Propranolol, Cardura®, Darvocet®, Tavist D®, oxybutynin, Axid®, Urecholine.

<u>Office Evaluation:</u>

Pelvic exam:	Grade I cystocele and rectocele
Q-tip test:	Resting angle = 6 degrees
	Valsalva angle = 66 degrees
	Angle change = 60 degrees
Stress test:	(cough) Instantly positive
Uro Flow:	Voided volume = 100 cc
	Postvoid volume = 10 cc

<u>Management:</u>   Bladder drills
                          Oxybutynin 2.5 mg TID
Consultation with internist to alter medications
  Urecholine—increases tone of detrusor producing a bladder contraction (patient was prescribed this to increase tone of pyloric sphincter).
  Oxybutynin—anticholinergic relaxes smooth muscle (decreased bladder contractions).
  Tavist®—antihistamine with anticholinergic and sedative side effects.
  Cardura®—alpha-blocker (may relax urethra).
  Propranolol—beta-blocker (may increase bladder tone).

<u>Follow-up:</u>

  Medications after adjustment:
    Synthroid®
    Premarin®
    Propranolol

"Patient states since her medications have been altered she is now perfectly dry and has never felt better. She is extremely happy."

CASE STUDY 2

<u>Profile:</u> 49-year-old white female P2002

<u>Chief Complaint:</u> Bladder spasms and incontinence

<u>History of Present Illness:</u> The patient notes urinary incontinence, frequency, and dribbling for four months. Urinary loss is in large amounts six times per day with laughter and position change. She soaks her clothing and the floor four to five times per day.

She urinates 8 to 19 times per day and has nocturia 4 to 5 times. She protects her bed with towels.

Office Evaluation:

Pelvic Exam:	Small Grade I cystocele and rectocele
	Appropriate soft-sharp sensations
Q-tip test:	Resting angle -5 degrees
	Valsalva angle $+1$ degree
	Change in angle 15 degrees
Stress test:	(Cough) negative
Uro Flow:	Voided volume 100 cc
	PVR 5 cc
Urodynamics:	Detrusor instability

Management:
> Oxybutynin 5 mg BID
> Estrogen vaginal cream

Follow-up:
> Patient satisfied with urination 8 to 10 times per day and no loss of urine.

CASE STUDY 3

Profile: 48-year-old P2002

Chief Complaint: Urinary incontinence and uterine bleeding

History of Present Illness: The patient has experienced urinary incontinence for one year, describing loss as small amounts several times a day. Leakage most often occurs with a full bladder associated with coughing, sneezing, laughing. She changes underwear three times per day. She also notes nocturia. She complains of prolonged and excessive menses associated with dysmenorrhea.

Surgeries: D&C for menometrorrhagia

Office Evaluation:

Pelvic exam:	Grade I cystocele
	Positive bulbocavernosus reflex
Q-tip:	Resting angle = 0 degree
	Valsalva angle = 60 degrees
	Change in angle = 60 degrees
Stress test:	(Cough) instantly positive
Uro Flow	Voided volume = 375 cc
	PVR = 40 cc
Urodynamics:	No detrusor contraction
	Maximum urethral closure pressure = 40 cm H_2O

Management:
Abdominal hysterectomy, bilateral salpingo oophorectomy, Burch retropubic urethropexy.

Follow-up: Continent

CASE STUDY 4

Profile: 44-year-old P4014

Chief Complaint: Urinary incontinence

History of Present Illness: The patient notes an 11-year history of urinary loss since the delivery of her last child. Urinary loss is in large amounts several times per day. Events that cause urinary loss include walking, washing dishes, dancing, and horseback riding. She wears a pad for protection and often cannot make it to the bathroom before leaking.

Surgeries: C-section × 1

Office Evaluation:

Pelvic exam:	Grade III cystocele and rectocele
	Positive bulbocavernosis reflex
Q-tip test:	Resting angle = 22 degrees
	Valsalva angle = 70 degrees
	Angle change = 48 degrees
Uro Flow:	Voided 15 cc; PVR = 10 cc
Urodynamics:	No detrusor instability
	Maximum urethral closure pressure = 28 cm H_2O
	Abdominal leak point pressure = >100 cm H_2O
Management:	Tension-free vaginal tape
	Anterior and posterior repair
Follow-up:	Continent

REFERENCES

1. Abrams P, Cardozo L, Fall M et al. Standardisation Sub-Committee of the International Continence Society. The standardisation of terminology in lower urinary tract function: Report from the Standardisation Sub-committee of the International Continence Society. Urol 2003; 61:37–49.
2. Hu TW, Wagner TH, Bentkover JD et al. Costs of urinary incontinence and overactive bladder in the United States: A comparative study. Urol 2004; 63:461–465.
3. Minassian VA, Drutz HP, Al-Badr A. Urinary incontinence as a worldwide problem. Int J Gynecol Obstet 2003; 82:327–338.
4. Harrison GL, Memel DS. Urinary incontinence in women: its prevalence and its management in a health promotion clinic. Br J Gen Pract 1994; 44(381):149–152.
5. Novielli KD, Simpson Z, Hua G et al. Urinary incontinence in primary care: a comparison of older African-American and Caucasian women. Int Urol Nephrol 2003; 35(3):423–428.
6. Holyrode-Ledue JM, Straus SE. Management of urinary incontinence in women. JAMA 2004; 291:986–995.
7. Viktrup L, Lose G, Rolff M et al. The symptom of stress incontinence caused by pregnancy or delivery in primiparas. Obstet Gynecol 1992; 79:945–949.
8. Arya LA, Jackson ND, Myers DL et al. Risk of new-onset urinary incontinence after forceps and vacuum delivery in primiparous women. Am J Obstet Gynecol 2001; 185:1318–1323.
9. Sampselle CM, Harlow SD, Skurnick J et al. Urinary incontinence predictors and life impact in ethnically diverse perimenopausal women. Obstet Gynecol 2002; 100:1230–1238.
10. Graham CA, Mallett VT. Race as a predictor of urinary incontinence and pelvic organ prolapse. Am J Obstet Gynecol 2001; 185:116–120.

11. Dallosso HM, Matthews RJ, McGrother CW et al. Leicestershire MRC Incontinence Study Group. The association of diet and other lifestyle factors with overactive bladder and stress incontinence: a longitudinal study in women. BJU Int 2003; 92:69–77.

12. Arya LA, Myers DL, Jackson ND. Dietary caffeine intake and the risk for detrusor instability: a case-control study. Obstet Gynecol 2000; 96(1):85–89.

13. Hextall AS, Majid L, Cardozo K. A prospective study of urinary symptoms in women with severe anorexia nervosa. Neurourol Urodyn 1999; 18:398–399.

14. Bo K, Borgen JS. Prevalence of stress and urge urinary incontinence in elite athletes and controls. Med Sci Sports Exer 2001; 33:1797–1802.

15. Bump RC, McClish DK. Cigarette smoking and urinary incontinence in women. Am J Obstet Gynecol 1992; 167:1213–1218.

16. Jiang K, Novi JM, Darnell S et al. Exercise and urinary incontinence in women. Obstet Gynecol Survey 2004; 59:717–721.

17. Davis G, Goodman M. Stress urinary incontinence in nulliparous female soldiers in airborne infantry training. J Pelv Surg 1996; 2:68–71.

18. Resnick NM. Urinary incontinence in older adults. Hosp Pract 1992; 27(10):139–142.

19. Caputo RM, Benson JT. The Q-tip test and urethrovesical junction mobility. Obstet Gynecol 1993; 82(6):892–896.

20. Summitt RL Jr, Sipes DR 2nd, Bent AE et al. Evaluation of pressure transmission ratios in women with genuine stress incontinence and low urethral pressure: A comparative study. Obstet Gynecol 1994; 83(6):77–81.

21. Pajoncini C, Costantini E, Guercini F et al. Clinical and urodynamics features of intrinsic sphincter deficiency. Neurourol Urodyn 2003; 22:264–268.

22. Van Brummen HJ, Heintz APM, van der Vaart CH. The association between overactive bladder symptoms and objective parameters from bladder diary and filling cystometry. Neurourol Urodyn 2004; 23:38–42.

23. Sutherland SE, Goldman HB. Treatment options for female urinary incontinence. Med Clin North Amer 2004; 88(2):96–110.

24. Tancer ML. The post-hysterectomy (vault) vesicovaginal fistula. J Urol 1980; 123:839–840.

25. Tancer ML. Observations on prevention and management of vesicovaginal fistula after total hysterectomy. Surg Gynecol Obstet 1992; 175:501–506.

26. Lee RA, Symmonds RE, Williams TJ. Current status of genitourinary fistula. Obstet Gynecol 1988; 72:313–319.

27. Smith GL, Williams G. Vesicovaginal fistula. BJU Int 1999; 83:564–570.

28. Lawson J. Tropical obstetrics and gynaecology III. Vesicovaginal fistula: a tropical disease. Trans R Soc Trop Med Hyg 1989; 83:454.

29. Wyman JF, Choi SC, Harkins SW et al. The urinary diary in evaluation of incontinent women: a test-retest analysis. Obstet Gynecol 1988; 71:812.

30. Baden WF, Walker TA, Lindsey JH. The vaginal profile. Tex Med 1968; 64(5):56–58.

31. Bump RC, Mattiasson A, Bo K et al. The standardization of terminology of female pelvic organ prolapse and pelvic floor dysfunction. Am J Obstet Gynecol 1996; 175(1):10–17.

32. Fantl JA, Newman DK, Colling J. Urinary incontinence in adults: acute and chronic management. Clinical Practice Guideline No. 2, 1996 Update (AHCPR Publication No. 96–0682). Rockville, MD: US Department of Health and Human Services, Public Health Service, Agency for Health Care Policy and Research; March 1996.

33. Culligan PJ, Heit M. Urinary incontinence in women: evaluation and management. Am Fam Physician 2000; 62:2433–2444.

34. Wilson ML, Gaido L. Laboratory diagnosis of urinary tract infections in adult patients. CID 2004; 38:1150–1158.

35. Koonings PP, Bergman A, Ballard CA. Low urethral pressure and stress urinary incontinence in women: risk factor for failed retropubic surgical procedure. Urol 1990; 36:245.

36. Nygaard I. Prevention of exercise incontinence with mechanical devices. J Reprod Med 1995; 40(2):89–94.

37. Robert M, Mainprize TC. Long-term assessment of the incontinence ring pessary for the treatment of stress incontinence. Int Urogynecol J Pelvic Floor Dysfunct 2002; 13(5): 326–329.
38. Aksac B, Aki S, Karan A et al. Biofeedback and pelvic floor exercises for the rehabilitation of urinary stress incontinence. Gynecol Obstet Invest 2003; 56(1):23–27.
39. Mouritsen L, Frimodt-Moller C, Moller M. Long-term effect of pelvic floor exercises on female urinary incontinence. Br J Urol 1991; 68:32–37.
40. Goode PS, Burgio KL, Locher JL et al. The effect of behavioral training with or without pelvic floor electrical stimulation on stress incontinence in women: a randomized controlled trial. JAMA 2003; 290:345–352.
41. Fantl JA, Cardozo L, McClish DK. Estrogen therapy in the management of urinary incontinence in postmenopausal women: a meta-analysis. First report of the Hormones and Urogenital Therapy Committee. Obstet Gynecol 1994; 83(1):23–32.
42. Robinson D, Cardozo L. Urogenital effects of hormone therapy. Best Pract Res Clin Endocrin Metab 2003; 17(1):91–104.
43. Grodstein F, Lifford K, Resnick NM et al. Postmenopausal hormone therapy and risk of developing urinary incontinence. Obstet Gynecol 2004; 103(2):254–260.
44. Bhatia NN, Bergman A, Karram MM. Effects of estrogen on urethral function in women with urinary incontinence. Am J Obstet Gynecol 1989; 160:176–181.
45. Tamussino KF, Zivkovic F, Pieber D et al. Five-year results after anti-incontinence operations. Am J Obstet Gynecol 1999; 181(6):1347–1352.
46. Drouin J, Tessier J, Bertrand PE et al. Burch colposuspension: long-term results and review of published reports. Urol 1999; 54:808–814.
47. Ou CS, Rowbotham R. Five-year follow-up of laparoscopic bladder neck suspension using synthetic mesh and surgical staples. J Laparoendosc Adv Surg Tech A 1999; 9(3):249–252.
48. Ulmsten U, Petros P. Intravaginal slingplasty (IVS): an ambulatory surgical procedure for treatment of female urinary incontinence. Scand J Urol Nephrol 1995; 29(1):75–82.
49. Sand PK, Winkler H, Blackhurst DW et al. A prospective randomized study comparing modified Burch retropubic urethropexy and suburethral sling for the treatment of genuine stress incontinence with low-pressure urethra. Am J Obstet Gynecol 2000; 182:30–34.
50. Rardin CR, Kohli N, Rosenblatt PL et al. Tension-free vaginal tape: outcomes among women with primary versus recurrent stress urinary incontinence. Obstet Gynecol 2002; 100:893–897.
51. Karram MM, Segal JL, Vassallo BJ et al. Complications and untoward effects of the tension-free vaginal tape procedure. Obstet Gynecol 2003; 101:929–932.
52. Meschia M, Pifarotti P, Bernasconi F et al. Tension-free vaginal tape: analysis of outcomes and complications in 404 stress incontinent women. Int Urogynecol J Suppl 2001; 2:S24–S27.
53. Croak AJ, Schulte V, Peron S et al. Transvaginal tape lysis for urinary obstruction after tension-free vaginal tape placement. J Urol 2003; 169:2238–2241.
54. deTayrac R, Deffieux X, Droupy S et al. A prospective randomized trial comparing tension-free vaginal tape and transobturator suburethral tape for surgical treatment of stress urinary incontinence. Am J Obstet Gynecol 2004; 190(3):602–608.
55. Fritel X, Zabak K, Pigne A et al. Predictive value of urethral mobility before suburethral tape procedure for urinary stress incontinence in women. J Urol 2002; 168:2472–2475.
56. Blavias JG. Pubovaginal sling. In: Kursh ED, McGuire EJ (eds). Female Urology. Philadelphia: J.B. Lippincott Company; 1994:239–249.
57. McGuire EJ, Lyttin B, Kohorn EL. Stress urinary incontinence. Obstet Gynecol 1976; 47: 255–264.
58. Chin YK, Stanton SL. A follow-up of silastic sling for genuine stress incontinence. Br J Obstet Gynaecol 1995; 102:143–147.
59. Morgan JE, Farrow GA, Stewart FE. The marlex sling operation for the treatment of recurrent stress urinary incontinence. A 16-year review. Am J Obstet Gynecol 1985; 151:224–226.
60. Summitt RL, Bent AE, Ostergaard DR et al. Suburethral sling procedure for genuine stress incontinence and low urethral closure pressure. Int Urogynecol J 1992; 3:18–21.

61. Pickard R, Reaper J, Wyness L et al. Periurethral injection therapy for urinary incontinence in women (Cochrane Review). In: Cochrane Library, Issue 1. Chichester, England: John Wiley and Sons; 2003.

62. Fantl JA, Wyman JF, McClish DK et al. Efficacy of bladder training in older women with urinary incontinence. JAMA 1991; 265:609–613.

63. Tapp AJ, Cardozo LD, Versi E et al. The treatment of detrusor instability in postmenopausal women with oxybutynin hydrochloride: a double-blind placebo-controlled study. Br J Obstet Gynaecol 1990; 97:521–526.

64. Moore KH, Hay DM, Imrie AE et al. Oxybutynin hydrochloride in the treatment of women with idiopathic detrusor instability. Br J Urol 1990; 66:479–485.

65. Appell RA, Sand P, Dmochowski R et al. Overactive Bladder: Judging Effective Control and Treatment Study Group. Prospective randomized controlled trial of extended-release oxybutynin chloride and tolterodine tartrate in the treatment of overactive bladder: results of the OBJECT study. Mayo Clin Proc 2001; 76:358–363.

66. Chapple C. Tolterodine once-daily: selectivity for the bladder over effects on salivation compared to Ditropan XL. J Urol 2001; 165:253.

67. Lee JG, Hong JY, Choo MS et al. Tolterodine: effective but better tolerated than oxybutynin in Asian patients with symptoms of overactive bladder. Int J Urol 2002; 9:247–252.

68. Abrams P, Freeman R, Anderstrom C et al. Tolterodine, a new antimuscarinic agent: as effective but better tolerated than oxybutynin in patients with overactive bladder. Br J Urol 1998; 8:801–810.

69. Dmochowski RR, Sand PK, Zinner Nr et al. Trospium 60 mg once daily (QD) for overactive bladder syndrome: results from a placebo-controlled intervention study. Urology 2008; 71(3):449–454.

70. Haab F, Corcos J, Siama P et al. Long-term treatment with darifenacin for overactive bladder: results of a two-year, open-label extension study. BJU Int 2006; 98(5):1025–1032.

71. Chapple CR, Cardozo L, Steers WD et al. Solifenacin significantly all symptoms of overactive bladder syndrome. Int J Clin Pract 2006; 60(8):959–966.

72. Barroso JC, Ramos JG, Martins-Costa S et al. Transvaginal electrical stimulation in the treatment of urinary incontinence. BJU Int 2004; 93:319–323.

73. Vandoninck V, van Balken MR, Finazzi Agro E et al. Percutaneous tibial nerve stimulation in the treatment of overactive bladder: urodynamics data. Neurourol Urodyn 2003; 22:227–232.

74. Almeida FG, Bruschini H, Srougi M. Urodynamic and clinical evaluation of 91 female patients with urinary incontinence treated with perineal magnetic stimulation: 1-year follow-up. J Urol 2004; 171:1571–1575.

75. Schmidt RA, Jonas U, Oleson KA et al. Sacral nerve stimulation for the treatment of refractory urinary urge incontinence. J Urol 1999; 162:352–357.

76. Weil EH, Ruiz-Cerda JL, Erdmans PH et al. Sacral nerve root neuromodulation in the treatment of refractory urinary urge incontinence: a prospective randomized clinical trial. Eur Urol 2000; 37:161–171.

77. Andersson KE, Appell R, Cardozo LD et al. The pharmacological treatment of urinary incontinence. BJU Int 1999; 84:923–947.

78. Paick JS, Ku JH, Kim SW et al. Tension-free vaginal tape procedure for the treatment of mixed urinary incontinence: significance of maximal urethral closure pressure. J Urol 2004; 172(3):1001–1005.

79. Osman T. Stress incontinence surgery for patients with mixed incontinence and a normal cystometrogram. BJU Int 2003; 92(9):964–968.

80. Novi JM, Rose M, Shaunik A et al. Conservative management of vesicouterine fistula after uterine rupture. Int Urogyn J Pelvic Floor Dysfunct 2004; 15(6):328–330.

81. Davits RJ, Miranda SI. Conservative treatment of vesicovaginal fistulas by bladder drainage alone. Br J Urol 1991; 68(2):155–156.

9

Pelvic Organ Prolapse in the Perimenopausal Patient

Gina M. Northington and Emily Saks
Department of Obstetrics and Gynecology, University of Pennsylvania, Philadelphia, Pennsylvania, U.S.A.

I. INTRODUCTION

Pelvic organ prolapse (POP) is the protrusion or herniation of pelvic structures such as the bladder, bowel, or uterus into the vaginal canal resulting from weakness or damage to the pelvic support structures. It may be associated with pelvic discomfort as well as sexual, urinary, and defecatory disorders. As many as 50% of adult women over the age of 40 are affected by pelvic organ prolapse and both the incidence and prevalence are known to increase with age (1,2). Additionally, a woman carries an 11% lifetime risk of undergoing an operation for prolapse or urinary incontinence by age 80 (3). Many women have signs of pelvic floor weakness and pelvic organ prolapse during routine gynecological examination (4). In a multicenter observational study done in the United States, the prevalence of pelvic organ prolapse among women aged 18 to 83 with stage I or greater was 76% and there was a 38% increased risk of POP with each advancing decade of age (1). In the past, prolapse was described by the structures perceived to be located behind the vaginal bulge such as cystocele, rectocele, or enterocele (Table 1). The use of these terms has been discouraged as it is not always certain which organs truly exist in the bulge. The affected vaginal segment, such as anterior or posterior wall prolapse, vault or uterine prolapse or perineal descent has recently been advocated to describe pelvic organ prolapse (5).

Accordingly, pelvic organ prolapse is becoming a more common diagnosis among perimenopausal women, resulting in an increased need for pelvic floor dysfunction services. Although not a life-threatening condition, pelvic organ prolapse can cause distressing pelvic floor symptoms, lead to a decreased quality of life, and withdrawal from social activity (6,7).

Table 1 Types of Pelvic Organ Prolapse

Disease	Characteristics	Vaginal segment
Cystocele	• Downward displacement of the bladder (anterior vaginal wall)	Anterior prolapse
Cystourethrocele	• May be associated with marked urethral hypermobility	Anterior prolapse
Uterine/vaginal vault prolapse	• Descent of the uterus or vaginal vault through the length of the vaginal canal	Apical prolapse
Rectocele	• Protrusion of the rectum/posterior vaginal wall into the vaginal canal	Posterior prolapse—may also be associated with perineal descent
Enterocele	• Herniation of small bowel into the lumen of the vagina • A catheter placed in the bladder may distinguish a cystocele from an anterior enterocele	May be a component of anterior, posterior, or apical prolapse

II. RISK FACTORS

The precise etiology of pelvic organ prolapse is not clear but is believed to be multi-factorial. Childbirth, operative vaginal delivery, and increasing parity are considered to be the strongest risk factors for the development of prolapse (2,8). Prolapse is often related to the stretch, pressure, and neuromuscular trauma that is associated with labor and vaginal childbirth. Although less common, prolapse does occur in women who have not had children. This highlights the role of genetics and ethnicity in a woman's predisposition to develop prolapse (2,9). Increasing age and body mass index are also thought to be associated with an increased risk of pelvic organ prolapse (2,8). Additionally, conditions that increase intra-abdominal pressure such as chronic cough, chronic constipation (10) or heavy lifting (11) may increase the risk of developing pelvic organ prolapse. Prior hysterectomy has also been implicated presumably because the vaginal vault was not reattached to the uterosacral and cardinal ligament complex at the time of hysterectomy (12).

It is helpful to organize risk factors in the following categories: predisposing, inciting, promoting, and decompensating (13). As noted in Table 2, some factors overlap categories. Although predisposing factors such as race, genetics, disorders of collagen synthesis, and structure, as well as congenital neuromuscular disorders have been associated with an increased risk of prolapse, there is no current method to screen normal individuals for those that will go on to develop symptomatic POP. Potentially modifiable risk factors are mode of delivery, obesity, chronic constipation, prior pelvic surgery, smoking, and estrogen depletion. However, modification of one or more risk factors has not been shown to significantly reduce the incidence of this disorder. This suggests that POP probably results from the complex interactions of multiple factors.

A. Pathogenesis

Anatomically, pelvic organ support can be divided into two categories: Levator ani complex (pelvic floor skeletal muscles) and endopelvic fascia (Fig. 1). The pelvic floor is

Table 2 Risk Factors for Pelvic Organ Prolapse

Predisposing	Inciting	Promoting	Decompensating
Gender	Vaginal childbirth	Constipation	Aging
Race/ethnicity	Neuromuscular injury	Occupation	Disability
Neurologic disorders	Radiation exposure	Obesity	Disease
Muscular dystrophy	Radical surgery	Pelvic surgery	Environment
Environmental	Pregnancy	Lung disease	Dementia
Genetics		Smoking	
		Infection	
		Menopause	

Source: Ref. 13.

made up of the levator ani and coccygeus muscles. The levator ani has three parts including the puborectalis, pubococcygeus, and iliococcygeus muscles. These muscles create a hammock between the pubis and coccyx, attaching laterally along the pelvic sidewalls. The levator ani muscle is tonically contracted, providing a firm shelf posteriorly to support the pelvic contents and aiding with urinary and fecal continence. If the levator ani muscles lose tone or are directly injured, the genital hiatus is enlarged and the prior shelf of support for the pelvic organs is removed (5). The endopelvic fascia is a loose network of connective tissue that surrounds and supports the pelvic organs and vagina. Condensations of the endopelvic fascia are known as the uterosacral and cardinal ligaments and the rectovaginal and vesicovaginal septum. These condensations help to keep the vagina in its normal position in the pelvis, directed posteriorly toward the sacrum (14). Tension or tearing of the endopelvic fascia can result in repositioning of the pelvic organs. Weakened levator ani and endopelvic fascia, together, lead to an enlarged genital hiatus and pelvic organ prolapse.

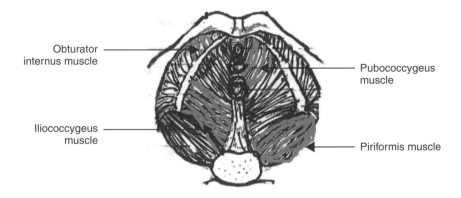

Figure 1 Levator ani muscles.

Our understanding of pelvic anatomy is augmented by considering the vagina as having three levels of support (Fig. 2). The apex (level I) is supported by the cardinal and uterosacral ligaments and failure results in uterine prolapse or vault prolapse post-hysterectomy. The midvagina (level II) is supported by the attachment of the vagina to the levator ani at the arcus tendineus fascia pelvis (white line) and failure results in a cystocele or rectocele. The lower vagina (level III) is supported by its attachment to the perineal membrane and perineal body. Failure at any one or more of these levels will result in a relaxed vaginal outlet and promote pelvic organ prolapse (15).

B. Pelvic Organ Prolapse in Perimenopause

Menopause is one of the more controversial risk factors for pelvic organ prolapse. Several studies have indicated that POP increases with age (1,2,4); however, it is unclear if estrogen depletion or the aging process leading to a degeneration of fibromuscular tissue is the cause of the anatomic and functional defects associated with POP. There is some evidence that women in the perimenopausal period have an increased incidence of POP. Samuelsson et al. (1999) performed a cross-sectional study of 641 women aged 20 to 59 from a primary health care district in Sweden and showed that women in the perimenopausal age

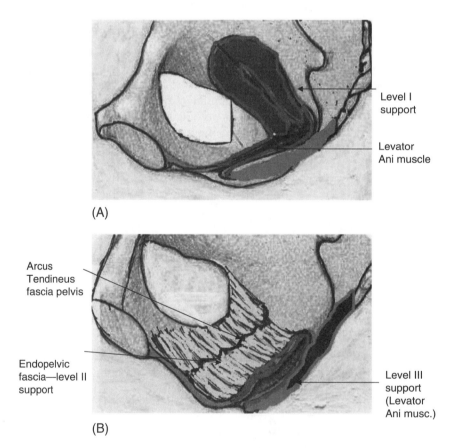

Figure 2 (A) Level I and level III support (B) level II and level III support—endopelvic fascia in light shaded region.

group (40 to 59 years) had a higher prevalence of POP (45% to 55%) when compared with younger women (4). These findings of an increased risk of POP in the perimenopausal period have been confirmed by others examining women in a similar age range (1). Accordingly, Luber et al. (2001) showed a comparable rate of consultation for pelvic organ prolapse across age ranges in women aged 30 to 89 indicating that younger peri-menopausal women are equally likely to develop significant symptoms associated with POP as compared to older women (16). Lang et al. (2003) noted that lower serum estra-diol levels and estrogen receptor values in the uterosacral ligaments of premenopausal women were significantly associated with pelvic organ prolapse (17). Although, estrogen replacement has been shown to increase total skin collagen content (18) and the matura-tion index of vaginal epithelial cells (19), there is no evidence that treating peri- or postmenopausal women with estrogen reduces the risk or severity of pelvic organ prolapse. In fact, results from the Women's Health Initiative (WHI) study did not demonstrate a reduction in the incidence of POP in postmenopausal women treated with HRT for six years (2). However, HRT may decrease the need for surgery for pelvic floor disorders (including pelvic organ prolapse) probably as a result of symptom improvement from asso-ciated pelvic floor disorders (20).

C. Evaluation

1. History

Many women with mild prolapse are asymptomatic. Advanced forms of prolapse may prompt patients to report feeling or seeing a bulge of vaginal tissue, experiencing pelvic pressure, or a feeling of a mass in the vagina. The report of feeling a bulge or that some-thing is falling out of the vagina has been shown to have a positive and negative predictive value for prolapse of 81% and 76%, respectively (21). Patients may also describe bother-some symptoms of pelvic floor dysfunction including urinary or fecal incontinence or dif-ficulties with urinating or defecating, necessitating digital assistance to void or evacuate the rectum (22). Specific questions to ask patients with POP about their pelvic floor func-tion are shown in Table 3. Urinary splinting—or the need to valsalva or assist with void-ing which may indicate bladder outlet obstruction—had 97% specificity for anterior prolapse. Ellerkman et al. (2001) also showed that urinary dysfunction including the need to change positions to empty was moderately associated with severe anterior and apical prolapse (22). However, symptoms associated with defecatory dysfunction including dig-ital assistance with defecation and obstructed defecation have not been shown to correlate with the severity or location of POP defects (21,22).

Patients may also report poor sexual functioning or less frequent sexual activity with the presence of prolapse (23). An increasing grade of prolapse has been associated with an interference with sexual activity (24) and women with POP may be more likely to report an absence of libido, lack of sexual excitement, and lack of orgasm (p < 0.05) (25). However, no correlation with sexual satisfaction and severity of prolapse has been shown (26). Therefore, if a patient is sexually active, it is important to gather information about pain during intercourse, problems with penetration, and if the patient has been having sexual intercourse less often.

Pelvic organ prolapse often coexists with urinary incontinence and fecal inconti-nence. Symptoms of stress urinary incontinence, urge urinary incontinence, urinary fre-quency, and urgency are associated with POP (27). A proposed mechanism for stress urinary incontinence in the setting of pelvic organ prolapse is through higher urethral pressure transmission (28). However, since most women have mixed urinary symptoms,

Table 3 Questions for Patients with Pelvic Organ Prolapse

Pelvic organ dysfunction	Specific questions
Urinary dysfunction	• Is there difficulty initiating a urinary stream (hesitancy)? • Do you have to manually push the bladder to initiate stream or completely empty? • Do you often switch positions or bear down to complete urination? • Do you have recurrent urinary tract infections? • Is there urinary incontinence?
Defecatory dysfunction	• Do you have fecal incontinence? Incontinence of flatus or stool? • Do you use your fingers to help with a bowel movement? • Do you have frequent constipation/diarrhea? • Do you have painful defecation?
Sexual function	• Are you sexually active? • Do you have pain during intercourse? • Is penetration a problem during intercourse? • Do you have intercourse less often and if so, why?

a thorough history and use of a validated questionnaire will help identify the specific type of urinary incontinence (29). Fecal incontinence may also coexist with pelvic organ prolapse but a specific relationship has not been demonstrated in the literature (30). This symptom may result from anal sphincter defects and pelvic floor neuropathy which often result from a complicated vaginal delivery—a recognized risk factor of POP. During the history, it is important to identify specific symptoms associated with prolapse as they may require alternative or adjunctive therapy to optimize patient satisfaction with treatment.

2. Physical Examination

In the perimenopausal patient, physical assessment should include a detailed general medical and pelvic examination consisting of inspection of the external and internal genitalia and bimanual examination. During a detailed medical examination, any signs of disorders that may lead to increased intra-abdominal pressure including chronic obstructive pulmonary disease, increased abdominal circumference from obesity or congestive heart failure, or signs of neuromuscular disease such as reflex abnormalities or diffuse muscle atrophy should be documented.

During the pelvic exam, the physician should focus on the location and severity of prolapse. It is also important that the patient be examined in both the lithotomy and standing position to evaluate the maximal descent of the prolapse (31,32). The severity of prolapse can be easily graded using the Baden-Walker Staging System for pelvic organ prolapse (Table 4) (33). However, the International Continence Society recently developed a more detailed grading system called the pelvic organ prolapse quantification (POP-Q) System that is used more often in research and the published literature (Tables 5 and 6) (34,35). The POP-Q system has also demonstrated strong inter- and intraobserver agreement (36). For clinical purposes, it is probably more important to be consistent by using the same staging system in order to track disease progression or response to treatment over time.

Table 4 Baden-Walker Staging System for POP

Grade	Location of leading structure[a]
0	No descent[b]
1	Maximal descent halfway to the hymenal ring
2	Maximal descent to the hymen
3	Maximal descent past the hymen—retracts above the hymen at rest
4	Maximal descent past the hymen—no retraction above the hymen at rest

[a]Leading structure usually relates to the specific organ that is prolapsed (i.e., bladder, urethra, cervix/vaginal cuff) or may be applied to the posterior cul-de-sac or perineal body.
[b]Descent is defined as using relationship of structures to ischial spines and hymenal ring
Source: Ref. 33.

Table 5 Pelvic Organ Prolapse Quantification System

Point	Anatomical correlation	Numerical range (cm)	Clinical diagnosis
Aa	Position of the midline anterior vagina 3 cm proximal to the external urethral meatus	−3 to +3	Anterior vaginal wall prolapse, cystocele, and/or anterior enterocele
Ba	Represents the most distal/most dependent point on the anterior vaginal wall from the vaginal cuff to point Aa	> −3	Anterior vaginal wall prolapse, cystocele, and/or anterior enterocele
C	The most distal/dependent edge of the cervix or leading edge of the vaginal cuff (after hysterectomy)	±TVL	Uterine or apical prolapse
D	Measurement of the level of uterosacral ligament attachment to the proximal posterior cervix. Measured in women with a cervix in place	±TVL	Uterine prolapse (may also suggest presence of high enterocele)
Ap	Position of the midline of the posterior vaginal wall 3 cm proximal to the hymen	−3 to +3	Posterior vaginal wall prolapse, rectocele, and/or enterocele
Bp	Represents the most distal/most dependent point on the posterior vaginal wall from the vaginal cuff to point Ap	> −3	Posterior vaginal wall prolapse, rectocele, and/or enterocele
GH	Vertical length of the genital hiatus measured from the middle of the external urethral meatus to the posterior midline of the hymen	Varies	May correlate with severity of pelvic organ prolapse
PB	Measured from the posterior margin of the genital hiatus to the mid-anal opening	Varies	Identifies perineal defect
TVL	Total vaginal length when point C and D are reduced to normal position	Varies	

Table 6 International Continence Society Pelvic Organ Prolapse Staging System

Stage	Characteristics
Stage 0	Points Aa, Ap, Ba, and Bp are all at –3 cm and either point C or D is at no more than –(TVL–2) cm
Stage I	The criteria for stage 0 are not met and the leading edge of prolapse is less than –1 cm
Stage II	Leading edge of prolapse is at least –1 cm but no more than +1 cm
Stage III	Leading edge of prolapse is greater than +1 cm but less than +(TVL – 2) cm
Stage IV	Leading edge of prolapse is at least +(TVL – 2) cm

Refer to Table 4 for definition of points (Aa, Ap, Ba, Bp, C, and D) and lengths (TVL: Total vaginal length).
Source: Ref. 34.

Another important aspect of the physical exam is a detailed neuromuscular examination to assess sensory, muscle strength, and reflexes associated with the pudendal nerve. Recurrent trauma to the pudendal nerves can occur during perineal descent, and can lead to denervation and weakness of the external anal sphincter muscle (37). This may be as a result from straining due to chronic constipation or from prolonged pushing during vaginal delivery. Digital assessment of pelvic floor contractions strength is also important and shows good agreement with vaginal perineometry and should be documented as part of the examination (38).

The physician should inspect for signs of vaginal atrophy (erythema or loss of rugosity) to determine the strength and integrity of the underlying pubocervical and rectovaginal fascia. A rectal examination will further assess the integrity of the rectovaginal septum as well as the extent of a rectocele/enterocele, the central tendon of the perineal body, and the strength of anal sphincter tone. Similarly, the Q-tip test, which assesses the angle of a sterile cotton swab placed in the urethra with valsalva, can indicate urethral hypermobility (angle > 30°), and may be helpful for planning treatment of coincident urinary incontinence. Any patient complaining of symptoms associated with voiding dysfunction should have their post void residual (PVR) volume measured either by catheterization or bladder ultrasound immediately following a void to determine if there is bladder outlet obstruction.

3. Imaging

Currently there are no imaging methods required for the accurate diagnosis of pelvic organ prolapse. However, imaging studies may be employed if there are symptoms that are unexplained by findings on the physical exam or when there is severe pelvic floor dysfunction out of proportion to the severity of pelvic organ prolapse. One may also consider imaging studies in patients with pelvic organ prolapse recurrence following surgical repair. Magnetic resonance imaging (MRI) can visualize pelvic viscera and muscles and may be used to distinguish vaginal cysts from prolapse. Dynamic MRI has demonstrated a high sensitivity for cystocele, urethrocele, and uterovaginal prolapse (39). Pelvic ultrasound may be useful for examining the urethrovesical junction and anterior vaginal wall descent (40,41). Pelvic fluoroscopy may also be used to further evaluate enteroceles, sigmoidoceles, and rectoceles (42). Endoanal ultrasound will provide information regarding the integrity of the anal sphincter. However, given the lack of standard radiologic criteria for

POP, imaging is rarely used for the diagnosis of prolapse but may be more useful for providing objective measures in research.

D. Treatment

1. Nonsurgical Treatment

Recognizing that some degree of prolapse is exceedingly common in perimenopausal women (43), observation of prolapse in an asymptomatic patient is an acceptable option. The prognosis of asymptomatic prolapse in a specific patient is uncertain as it may progress or remain the same. Although there are no recognized lifestyle measures that conclusively alter the course of POP, it is reasonable to encourage healthy lifestyle changes such as diet, exercise, and smoking cessation that promote a healthy weight and strong fibromuscular tissue. However, the presence of prolapse on exam should prompt the physician to inquire about and evaluate for concomitant urinary or defecatory dysfunction, as this may be a reason to advise more aggressive treatment.

Physical therapy may be appropriate for symptoms of pelvic floor dysfunction that are associated with pelvic organ prolapse (44). There is some evidence that a program of pelvic floor muscle exercises may decrease the rate of worsening prolapse (45). However, there is no conclusive evidence that pelvic floor muscle exercises reduce the incidence of pelvic organ prolapse (46). Although expectant management is appropriate for POP, it is important to monitor women with advanced stages of POP for signs and symptoms of severe urinary obstruction, obstructive defecation, vaginal erosion, and significant hydronephrosis resulting from chronic ureteral kinking associated with vaginal eversion as these patients may require more invasive therapy.

For symptomatic prolapse, nonsurgical treatment can be attempted using a pessary. This is a flexible device made of plastic or silicone that is placed into the vagina to support prolapse (Fig. 3). There are a wide variety of pessaries and it should be selected based on the type and severity of prolapse along with the size of the genital hiatus (Table 7). The ring, gelhorn, and donut pessaries are the most frequently used (47). Although pessary use has been traditionally reserved for older patients that are not good candidates for pelvic reconstructive surgery, it should also be offered to symptomatic perimenopausal women who want to consider alternatives to surgery. Other indications for pessaries include their use as a temporizing measure while a patient is awaiting surgery or to aid in the preoperative healing of erosions in patients with massive prolapse. Pessaries are also useful as a preoperative diagnostic aid to assist in determining if a woman's pelvic discomfort or back pain is due to pelvic organ prolapse (48). While a pessary will not cure prolapse, in some cases a pessary may slow the progression of POP (49). Successful fitting includes matching pessary size with an individual patient and correcting symptoms associated with pelvic organ prolapse. During the fitting procedure, patients should be asked to perform the valsalva maneuver, walk, stand, and bend repetitively to make sure the pessary is not dislodged during normal activities. The physician should be able to easily remove the pessary by placing a finger between the pessary and vaginal wall. The patient should also be able to void and defecate without difficulty. Side effects of using a pessary include vaginal irritation, bleeding, discharge, or ulceration. Pessary use can sometimes result in urinary incontinence through the unmasking of underlying intrinsic sphincter deficiency. Worsening urinary incontinence has been associated with discontinuation of the pessary (50,51). Indeed, pessaries are associated with a high dropout rate of up to 50% after three years (50). In general, patients with pessaries in place should be seen at two- to three-month intervals

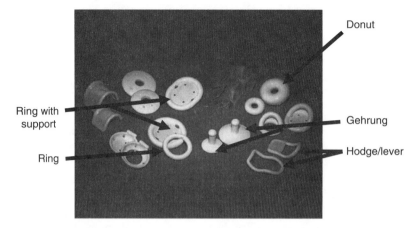

Figure 3 Pessary—various sizes and shapes. (Photo courtesy of Mentor Corp.)

Table 7 Pessary Selection and Management

Prolapse	Pessary[a]	Comment[b]
Uterine prolapse	Ring pessary	Fitting of this pessary is similar to the fitting of a contraceptive diaphragm. Patients can be taught self-care. Sexual activity is possible with pessary in place.
Cystocele	Ring with support pessary	The additional support prevents protrusion of a cystocele.
Apical prolapse, massive prolapse	Donut pessary	Vaginal intercourse is precluded. Frequent visits are required for removal, cleaning, and reinsertion.
Uterine prolapse, cystocele, and/or rectocele	Gehrung	This pessary can be manually molded to fit an individual patient—concavity downward for cystocele and uterine prolapse; concavity upward for rectocele. Intercourse is possible with the pessary in place.
Uterine prolapse	Lever pessaries (Hodge, Smith, and Risser)	Not designed for sexual intercourse while pessary is in place. Frequent office visits for pessary removal, cleaning, and reinsertion
Massive prolapse with poor perineal support	Cube pessary	This should be the pessary of last resort because of the high risk of severe vaginal erosion, bleeding, and infection. Patients cannot be taught self-care and vaginal intercourse is precluded.
Massive vault prolapse with poor muscle tone	Gellhorn	The concave surface of the pessary fits against the cervix or vaginal cuff with stem directed downward toward the perineal body. The stem prevents sexual intercourse. Most patients are unable to remove and care for this pessary at home and require frequent visits for pessary cleaning.

[a]Many patients do not have an isolated type of prolapse and may benefit from any of the available pessaries.
[b]Use of any pessary may cause vaginal ulceration or erosion, vaginal discharge, vaginal bleeding, and pain. The effects listed are most commonly associated with these effects.

and those with atrophic vaginitis should use a topical estrogen intravaginally to help prevent erosion. Patients who are able to remove and clean the pessary on their own will require less frequent follow-up and will be able to continue sexual activity. For the perimenopausal patient, pelvic floor function and goals of therapy should be used to individualize pessary selection for pelvic organ prolapse.

2. Surgical Treatment

Perimenopausal women who desire definitive surgical therapy or fail conservative therapy are candidates for surgical management of pelvic organ prolapse. Reconstructive surgical procedures aim to restore normal anatomic relationships in the pelvis while preserving or restoring pelvic floor function. The goal of surgical repairs should be to address all vaginal wall and pelvic muscle defects since isolated defects are uncommon (1,2). This approach often requires a combination of procedures which should be planned and discussed with patients at length preoperatively. The specific type and route of procedure depends on the site or extent of prolapse as well as the patient and surgeon's preferences. Although the vaginal approach to pelvic reconstructive surgery is commonly performed (3), in some cases it may be advisable to perform abdominal reconstructive procedures to correct POP.

Apical prolapse involves the failure of level I support and surgical therapy requires the reconstruction of this support mechanism at or near the apex of the vagina. Vaginal repair of apical prolapse most commonly involves the attachment of the vaginal apex or cervix to one or both of the sacrospinous ligaments. However, it may also be performed by suspending the vaginal apex to the iliococcygeus muscles or the uterosacral ligaments. The most commonly performed abdominal procedure for apical prolapse is the abdominal sacrocolpopexy that uses a mesh (usually synthetic) as a suspensory bridge between the vaginal apex and the sacral periosteum at the level of S3 or S4. This procedure has been associated with a lower rate of recurrent apical prolapse and postoperative dyspareunia as compared to vaginal sacrospinous suspension procedures in randomized controlled trials (52). Although this procedure is associated with a longer operating time, slower return to activities of daily living, and a greater cost as compared to vaginal procedures (52) it should be considered for young perimenopausal patients given its proven durability over time (53).

Performing a hysterectomy at the time of apical prolapse repair was once thought to be an important component of a successful repair. The reason for this is that the weight of the uterus was thought to impart excess tension leading to an increase rate of recurrent apical prolapse. However, there is no conclusive data to support this theory. Further, hysterectomy at the time of abdominal sacrocolpopexy is a known risk factor for mesh erosion (54). Alternatives to total hysterectomy at the time of abdominal sacrocolpopexy are supracervical hysterectomy and sacral mesh hysteropexy (55). Recently, other procedures that provide for uterine preservation have emerged including intravaginal slingplasty and laparoscopic uterosacral ligament plication. These procedures have demonstrated good short-term success rates (56,57). Perimenopausal patients who wish to maintain their reproductive organs have several options when undergoing an apical repair and the decision to perform a hysterectomy should be made on an individual basis.

Anterior wall prolapse is corrected by either colporrhaphy (plication of the vesicovaginal fascia in the midline) or paravaginal repair (reattachment of the lateral vagina to the arcus tendineus fascia pelvis) depending on the site of the defect. Paravaginal repairs can be approached either abdominally or vaginally. Although several retrospective trials have shown an 80 to 100% success rate of anterior colporrhaphy (58,59), more recent prospective randomized controlled trials comparing anterior repair procedures have reported lower success rates (40–50%) (60,61). Cure rates for vaginal paravaginal repair has been reported to be as high as 98% (62). Higher cure rates have been shown when vaginal paravaginal repair was augmented with graft material (63).

Posterior wall prolapse is usually repaired by either colporrhaphy (plication of the rectovaginal fascia/levator ani muscles in the midline) or site-specific repair (closing specific defects visualized in the rectovaginal fascia). Plication of the rectovaginal fascia and/or levator ani muscles in the midline may be associated with postoperative dyspareunia in up to 50% of patients (64). Alternatively, site-specific posterior repairs are associated with an 82% cure rate without a high rate of postoperative dyspareunia (65). It should be noted that anatomical reconstruction of posterior defects may not restore bowel function in patients with severe long-standing defecatory dysfunction (66). Therefore, individuals with significant bowel symptoms may require further work up by a colorectal surgeon before proceeding with pelvic surgery. Often, posterior defects that are accompanied by a relaxed vaginal outlet will require a concomitant perineorrhaphy—reapproximation of the transverse perineal and bulbocavernosus muscles—to complete the repair.

Because pelvic organ prolapse surgery may be associated with a reoperation rate of almost 30% (3), some surgeons have employed the use of an implant material—biologic or synthetic—to reinforce vaginal anterior or posterior repairs. However, there are few safety and efficacy trials found in the literature. In fact, up to 25% of cases have been associated mesh-related complications of which mesh erosion is the most common (67). Other adverse affects associated with mesh use include dyspareunia, chronic vaginal pain, and vaginal discharge (68–70). Severe complications may require reoperation to remove the mesh (71). Use of biologic materials (e.g., donor allograft or xenograft) have been advocated to reduce the incidence of mesh erosions. However, the data on the long-term functional and anatomical outcomes related to the use of these materials in pelvic reconstructive surgery is lacking (72,73). Presently, pelvic surgeons with experience using implant materials for pelvic reconstructive procedures should individualize the choice of materials to optimize pelvic floor function and prevent the occurrence of severe complications.

Obliterative surgical procedures are associated with a quicker operative time and less perioperative morbidity as compared to the previously mentioned reconstructive procedures. These procedures include total colpocleisis or LeFort's partial colpocleisis which correct POP by reducing or closing the vaginal canal and replacing pelvic organs into the pelvis (74,75). Although these procedures may be associated with improved quality of life in elderly women (76), they are rarely appropriate for young perimenopausal patients. This is because these procedures effectively eliminate the ability to engage in sexual intercourse and unless the uterus is removed, will prevent the adequate egress of menstrual and vaginal fluids in perimenopausal women. In rare cases of significant disability or comorbid conditions necessitating shorter operative times, obliterative procedures may be considered in the perimenopausal patient.

E. Prevention

There are no published successful prevention strategies for pelvic organ prolapse. It is reasonable to assume that lifestyle modifications such as smoking cessation, maintaining a normal BMI, treating chronic constipation, avoiding repetitive heavy lifting, and a healthy diet would reduce some of the inciting and promoting factors for POP. Additionally, avoiding risk factors related to vaginal delivery such as prolonged second stage of labor, delivery of a macrosomic infant, or operative vaginal delivery (e.g., use of forceps) would conceivably reduce the risk of POP. However, because there are also risks associated with cesarean section and especially repeat cesarean sections for subsequent deliveries, one should proceed with caution prior to making a general recommendation of elective cesarean section to prevent pelvic floor disorders. Further, most women who have had vaginal deliveries do not develop symptomatic POP (13) and pregnancy itself may be associated with the development of prolapse (77,78). More information is needed to develop effective risk reduction strategies that will prevent pelvic organ prolapse in women.

F. Recommendations for Subspecialty Referral

A consultation with a urologist, urogynecologist—a gynecologist who maintains a practice with a special emphasis on pelvic floor disorders, or a colorectal surgeon is recommended if the diagnosis of pelvic organ prolapse is unclear, if the patient has associated pelvic floor dysfunction (sexual, urinary, or defecatory), or if the patient desires surgical intervention. Functional disorders may require additional testing such as urodynamics, defecogram, pelvic endoscopy, anal manometry, and other pelvic imaging procedures that require expert interpretation and are useful for planning subsequent treatment. Often, the successful diagnosis and treatment of pelvic floor dysfunction requires a coordination of care between primary care physicians and pelvic surgeons in order to obtain optimal results for each patient.

III. SUMMARY

Pelvic organ prolapse is a common condition in perimenopausal women. Pelvic organ prolapse in the early stages with minimal symptoms does not require intervention. Watchful waiting is appropriate in these cases. However, in some women, POP will progress to a more severe stage and cause a reduction in their quality of life. Older women or perimenopausal women who do not desire surgery can be treated conservatively with pelvic floor muscle exercises and a pessary. Advanced prolapse or prolapse associated with significant pelvic floor disorders including lower urinary tract symptoms, defecatory dysfunction, or sexual disorders warrants referral to a specialist that can provide advanced treatment to address anatomical and functional disorders. Women often have a complex mix of symptoms related to pelvic floor function and therefore will benefit from a multidisciplinary approach to treatment.

CASE STUDY 1

Profile: 50-year-old female G3P2012

Chief Complaint: Prolapse

History of Present Illness: The patient had been seen for an annual gynecological exam and was told that her bladder and uterus had "dropped down." The patient denies exteriorized tissue, pelvic pressure, or pelvic pain. She reports urinating seven times per day and one time each night. She denies any urinary incontinence associated with coughing, sneezing, or urgency. She does report mild constipation that responds to a stool softener. She reports being sexually active with her partner without complaint.

Office Evaluation:

    Pelvic exam: Stage I cystocele and uterine prolapse

Q-tip test: 45 degrees
Stress test: Negative
Pelvic floor muscle strength: 3/5

Management: Expectant management recommended as this patient is asymptomatic. Counseling should include a discussion with the patient that in some women prolapse will progress although a time frame is unclear. Encourage a healthy diet, abstinence from smoking, and regular Kegel exercises to improve pelvic floor muscle strength.

Follow-up: Patient doing well with Kegel exercises plans to return for re-evaluation if the prolapse becomes symptomatic or if she develops any urinary or fecal complaints.

CASE STUDY 2

Profile: 48-year-old female G3P3003

Chief Complaint: Splinting with defecation and excessive menses

History of Present Illness: The patient reports having constipation despite use of stool softener and occasional laxatives. She also reports only being able to have a bowel movement once she pushes on her perineum in between her vaginal and rectal openings. She denies any fecal incontinence. She also reports very heavy menses, unresponsive to hormonal treatment and recently had an unremarkable pelvic ultrasound and normal pathology from a D&C. She denies any leakage of urine and is not currently in a sexual relationship.

Office Evaluation:

Pelvic exam:	Stage I cystocele
	Stage I uterine prolapse
	Stage III rectocele
Q-tip test:	50 degrees
Stress test:	Negative
Uro Flow:	Voided volume = 375 cc
	PVR = 40 cc
Urodynamics (done with POP reduced):	
	No detrusor contraction
	No leakage with cough or valsalva

Management: Patient offered a hysterectomy with rectocele repair given the menorrhagia and splinting with defecation. However, she was also referred to a colorectal surgeon for further evaluation of her defecatory dysfunction prior to surgical repair.

Follow-up: This patient was started on a new bowel regimen with the colorectal surgeon. She also began a pelvic floor rehabilitation program to strengthen her pelvic floor muscles. She eventually opted for surgery. Given the patient's age and goals for treatment, she underwent a supracervical hysterectomy, an abdominal sacrocolpopexy, an abdominal paravaginal repair, a vaginal posterior repair with graft, and a perineorrhaphy. These procedures should address most of the defects noted on physical examination and improve pelvic function.

Follow-up: Postoperatively, the patient was doing well and by 3 months, she was back to her usual activities. She denied any urinary incontinence. This patient still had complaints of bowel dysfunction but to a lesser degree when compared with preoperative function. She restarted the pelvic floor muscle rehabilitation program.

CASE STUDY 3

Profile: 45-year-old female G4P4004

Chief Complaint: Uterine prolapse

History of Present Illness: The patient notes exteriorized vaginal tissue and cervix, especially when exercising at the gym. She does report feeling a "bulge" in the vagina but denies pelvic pain. She reports urinating about six times per day and rarely at night. She states that she previously had a problem with urine leakage while exercising, but no longer notes any leakage with increased abdominal pressure or with urgency. She denies any problems with her bowels or with sexual intercourse.

Office Evaluation:

Pelvic Exam:	Grade III cystocele
	Grade III uterine prolapse
	Grade I rectocele.
Q-tip test:	70 degrees
Uro Flow:	Voided volume 300 cc
	PVR 10 cc
Urodynamics:	Leak with cough @ 225 cc
	Leak with valsalva @ 450 cc
	No detrusor instability

Management: The gold standard surgical procedure for apical (uterine or vaginal vault) prolapse, an abdominal sacrocolpopexy, was recommended given the patient's age, physical activity, and stage of prolapse. Hysterectomy with abdominal sacrocolpopexy is a durable repair with a low recurrence rate. The procedure is also associated with a low risk of complications. Abdominal paravaginal repair and synthetic midurethral sling were also recommended for the cystocele and stress urinary incontinence with hypermobility.

Follow-up: The patient elected for definitive surgical treatment and underwent the above recommended procedures. She is continent of urine and doing well postoperatively. She has no complaints of dyspareunia.

CASE STUDY 4

Profile: 65-year-old female GP2002

Chief Complaint: Prolapsed bladder and urinary incontinence

History of Present Illness: The patient reports pelvic pressure and feeling a bulge when using the bathroom. She also reports leakage of urine with coughing, sneezing, and while running to the bathroom. She urinates about 10 times per day and two or three times each night. She wears a thin pad that she usually changes once or twice throughout the day. She denies any constipation, loose stool, or fecal incontinence. She is married but is concerned about decreased frequency of sexual intercourse. She explains that she does not feel attractive with a bulge "down there" and is nervous about leaking urine and therefore has been avoiding intercourse.

Office Evaluation:

Pelvic exam:	Grade II cystocele
	Grade II uterine prolapse
Q-tip test:	60 degrees
Uro Flow:	Voided 200 cc; PVR = 5 cc
Urodynamics:	Clonic detrusor instability noted first @ 200 cc
	Leak with cough @ 150 cc
	Leak with valsalva @ 150 cc, 300 cc

Management: Patient offered pessary and pelvic floor rehabilitation versus definitive surgical treatment for prolapse and mixed incontinence. She is a good candidate for a synthetic midurethral sling and anterior colporrhaphy to treat the mixed incontinence and prolapse; although she was counseled that she might still require medical management of the urge incontinence postoperatively. Her decreased frequency of sexual intercourse was also discussed and it was felt that this might resolve once the prolapse was repaired and her body image improved.

Follow-up: She elected for surgical treatment and was doing well postoperatively. She reported being content and feeling more secure in her sexual relationship.

REFERENCES

1. Swift SE. The distribution of pelvic organ support in a population of female subjects seen for routine gynecologic health care. American Journal of Obstetrics and Gynecology 2000; 183:277–285.
2. Hendrix SL, Clark A, Nygaard IE et al. Pelvic organ prolapse in the Women's Health Initiative: gravity and gravidity. American Journal of Obstetrics and Gynecology 2002; 186:1160–1166.
3. Olsen AL, Smith VJ, Bergstrom JO et al. Epidemiology of surgically managed pelvic organ prolapse. Obstetrics and Gynecology 1997; 89:501–506.
4. Samuelsson EC, arne Victor FT, Tibblin G et al. Signs of genital prolapse in a Swedish population of women 20 to 59 years of age and possible related factors. American Journal of Obstetrics and Gynecology 1999; 180:299–305.
5. Lien KC, Mooney B, Delancey JO et al. Levator ani muscle stretch induced by simulated vaginal birth. Obstetrics and Gynecology 2004; 103:31–40.
6. Diegsu GA, Chaliha C, Salvatore S et al. The relationship of vaginal prolapse severity to symptoms and quality of life. BJOG 2005; 112:971–976.
7. Jelovsek JE, Barber MD. Women seeking treatment for advanced pelvic organ prolapse have decreased body image and quality of life. American Journal of Obstetrics and Gynecology 2006; 194:1455–1461.
8. Mant J, Painter R, Vessey M. Epidemiology of genital prolapse: observations from the Oxford Family Planning Association study. BJOG 1997; 104:579–585.
9. Buchsbaum GM, Duecy EE, Kerr LA et al. Pelvic organ prolapse in nulliparous women and their parous sisters. Obstetrics and Gynecology 2006; 108:1388–1393.
10. Spence-Jones C, Kamm MA, Henry MM et al. Bowel dysfunction: a pathogenic factor in uterovaginal prolapse and urinary stress incontinence. 1994; 101–152.

11. Jorgensen S, Hein HO, Gyntelberg F. Heavy lifting at work and risk of genital prolapse and herniated lumbar disc in assistant nurses. Occupational Medicine 1994; 44:47–49.

12. Cruikshank SH. Preventing posthysterectomy vaginal vault prolapse and enterocele during vaginal hysterectomy. American Journal of Obstetrics and Gynecology 1987; 156:1433–1440.

13. Bump RC, Norton PA. Epidemiology and natural history of pelvic floor dysfunction. Obstetrics and Gynecology Clinics of North America 1998; 25:723–746.

14. Delancey JO. The anatomy of the pelvic floor. Clinical Opinions in Obstetrics and Gynecology 1994; 6:313–316.

15. Delancey JO. Anatomic aspects of vaginal eversion after hysterectomy. American Journal of Obstetrics and Gynecology 1992; 166:1717–1728.

16. Luber KM, Boero S, Choe JY. The demographics of pelvic floor disorders: current observations and future projections. American Journal of Obstetrics and Gynecology 2001; 184:1496–1501.

17. Lang JH, Zhu L, Sun ZJ et al. Estrogen levels and estrogen receptors in patients with stress urinary incontinence and pelvic organ prolapse. International Journal of Gynaecology and Obstetrics 2003; 80:35–39.

18. Brincat M, Versi E, Moniz CF et al. Skin collagen changes in postmenopausal women receiving different regimens of estrogen therapy. Obstetrics and Gynecology 1987; 70:123–127.

19. Vardy MD, Lindsay R, Scotti RJ et al. Short-term urogenital effects of raloxifene, tamoxifen, and estrogen. American Journal of Obstetrics and Gynecology 2003; 189:81–89.

20. Moalli PA, Jones Ivy S, Meyn LA et al. Risk factors associated with pelvic floor disorders in women undergoing surgical repair. Obstetrics and Gynecology 2003; 101:869–874.

21. Tan JS, Lukacz ES, Menefee SA et al. San Diego Pelvic Floor Consortium. Predictive value of prolapse symptoms: a large database study. International Urogynecology Journal 2005; 16:203–209.

22. Ellerkmann RM, Cundiff GW, Melick CF et al. Correlation of symptoms with location and severity of pelvic organ prolapse. American Journal of Obstetrics and Gynecology 2001; 185:1332–1337.

23. Rogers RG, Villarreal A, Kammerer-Doak D et al. Sexual function in women with and without urinary incontinence and/or pelvic organ prolapse. International Journal of Gynaecology and Obstetrics 2001; 12:361–365.

24. Weber AM, Walters MD, Schover LR et al. Sexual function in women with uterovaginal prolapse and urinary incontinence. Obstetrics and Gynecology 1995; 85:483–487.

25. Ozel B, White T, Urwitz-Lane R et al. The impact of pelvic organ prolapse on sexual function in women with urinary incontinence. International Urogynecology Journal 2006; 17:14–17.

26. Pauls RN, Berman JR. Impact of pelvic floor disorders and prolapse on female sexual function and response. Urologic Clinics of North America 2002; 29:677–683.

27. Marinkovic SP, Stanton SL. Incontinence and voiding difficulties associated with prolapse. Journal of Urology 2004; 171:1021–1028.

28. Bump RC, Fantl JA, Hurt WG. The mechanism of urinary continence in women with severe uterovaginal prolapse: results of barrier studies. Obstetrics and Gynecology 1988; 72:291–295.

29. Rogers RG, Coates KW, Kammerer-Doak D et al. A short form of the Pelvic Organ Prolapse/Urinary Incontinence Sexual Questionnaire (PISQ-12). International Urogynecology Journal 2003; 14:164–168.

30. Jackson SL, Weber AM, Hull TL et al. Fecal incontinence in women with urinary incontinence and pelvic organ prolapse. Obstetrics and Gynecology 1997; 89:423–427.

31. Visco AG, Wei JT, McClure LA et al. Effects of examination technique modifications on pelvic organ prolapse quantification (POP-Q) results. International Urogynecology Journal 2003; 14:136–140.

32. Barber MD, Lambers A, Visco AG et al. Effect of patient position on clinical evaluation of pelvic organ prolapse. Obstetrics and Gynecology 2000; 96:18–22.

33. Baden WF, Walker TA, Lindsey JH. The vaginal profile. Texas Medicine 1968; 64:56–58.

34. Bump RC, Mattiasson A, Bø K et al. The standardization of terminology of female pelvic organ prolapse and pelvic floor dysfunction. American Journal of Obstetrics and Gynecology 1996; 175:10–17.

35. Muir TW, Stepp KJ, Barber MD. Adoption of the pelvic organ prolapse quantification system in peer-reviewed literature. American Journal of Obstetrics and Gynecology 2003; 189:1632–1635.

36. Hall AF, Theofrastous JP, Cundiff GW et al. Interobserver and intraobserver reliability of the proposed International Continence Society, Society of Gynecologic Surgeons, and American Urogynecologic Society pelvic organ prolapse classification system. American Journal of Obstetrics and Gynecology 1996; 175:1467–1470.

37. Kiff ES, Barnes PR, Swash M. Evidence of pudendal neuropathy in patients with perineal descent and chronic straining at stool. Gut 1984; 25:1279–1282.

38. Isherwood PJ, Rane A. Comparative assessment of pelvic floor strength using a perineometer and digital examination. BJOG 2000; 107:1007–1011.

39. Gousse AE, Barbaric ZL, Safir MH et al. Dynamic half fourier acquisition, single shot turbo spin-echo magnetic resonance imaging for evaluating the female pelvis. Journal of Urology 2000; 164:1606–1613.

40. Peschers U, Schaer G, Anthuber C et al. Changes in vesical neck mobility following vaginal delivery. Obstetrics and Gynecology 1996; 88:1001–1006.

41. Dietz HP, Haylen BT, Broome J. Ultrasound in the quantification of female pelvic organ prolapse. Ultrasound in Obstetrics and Gynecology 2001; 18:511–514.

42. Kelvin FM, Hale DS, Maglinte DD et al. Female pelvic organ prolapse: diagnostic contribution of dynamic cystoproctography and comparison with physical examination. American Journal of Roentgenology 1999; 173:31–37.

43. Nygaard I, Bradley C, Brandt D, Women's Health Initiative. Pelvic organ prolapse in older women: prevalence and risk factors. Obstetrics and Gynecology 2004; 104:489–497.

44. Swart AM, Hagerty J, Corstiaans A et al. Management of the very weak pelvic floor. Is there a point? International Urogynecology Journal 2002; 13:346–348.

45. Piya-Anant M, Therasakvichya S, Leelaphatanadit C et al. Integrated health research program for the Thai elderly: prevalence of genital prolapse and effectiveness of pelvic floor exercise to prevent worsening of genital prolapse in elderly women. Journal of the Medical Association of Thailand 2003; 86:509–515.

46. Harvey MA. Pelvic floor exercises during and after pregnancy: a systematic review of their role in preventing pelvic floor dysfunction. Journal of Obstetrics and Gynaecology of Canada 2008; 25:487–498.

47. Cundiff GW, Weidner AC, Visco AG. A survey of pessary use by members of the American Urogynecologic Society. Obstetrics and Gynecology 2000; 95:931–935.

48. American Urogynecologic Society. The Vaginal Pessary. Quarterly Report (3). 1991. Washington, D.C., American Urogynecolgic Society.

49. Handa VL, Jones M. Do pessaries prevent the progression of pelvic organ prolapse? International Urogynecology Journal 2002; 13:349–351.

50. Wu V, Farrell SA, Baskett TF et al. A simplified protocol for pessary management. Obstetrics and Gynecology 1997; 90:990–994.

51. Veronikis DK, Nichols DH, Wakamatsu MM. The incidence of low-pressure urethra as a function of prolapse-reducing technique in patients with massive pelvic organ prolapse (maximum descent at all vaginal sites). American Journal of Obstetrics and Gynecology 1997; 177:1305–1314.

52. Maher CF, Qatawneh AM, Dwyer PL et al. Abdominal sacral colpopexy or vaginal sacrospinous colpopexy for vaginal vault prolapse: a prospective randomized study. American Journal of Obstetrics and Gynecology 2004; 190:20–26.

53. Nygaard IE, McCreery R, Brubaker L et al. Abdominal sacrocolpopexy: a comprehensive review. Obstetrics and Gynecology 2004; 104:805–823.

54. Benson JT, Lucente V, McClellan E. Vaginal versus abdominal reconstructive surgery for the treatment of pelvic support defects: a prospective randomized study with long-term outcome evaluation. American Journal of Obstetrics and Gynecology 1996; 175:1418–1421.

55. Rahn DD, Marker AC, Corton MM et al. Does supracervical hysterectomy provide more support to the vaginal apex than total abdominal hysterectomy? American Journal of Obstetrics and Gynecology 2007; 197:650e1–4.

56. Neuman M, Lavy Y. Conservatin of the prolapsed uterus is a valid option: medium term results of a prospective comparative study with the posterior intravaginal slingoplasty operation. International Urogynecology Journal 2007; 18:889–893.

57. Uccella S, Ghezzi F, Bergamini V et al. Laparoscopic uterosacral ligaments plication for the treatment of uterine prolapse. Archives of Gynecology and Obstetrics 2007; 276:225–229.

58. Stanton SL, Hilton P, Norton C et al. Clinical and urodynamic effects of anterior colporrhaphy and vaginal hysterectomy for prolapse with and without incontinence. BJOG 1982; 89:459–463.

59. Porges RF, Smilen SW. Long-term analysis of the surgical management of pelvic support defects. American Journal of Obstetrics and Gynecology 1994; 171:1518–1526.

60. Weber AM, Walters MD, Piedmonte MR et al. Anterior colporrhaphy: a randomized trial of three surgical techniques. American Journal of Obstetrics and Gynecology 2001; 185:1299–1304.

61. Sand PK, Koduri S, Lobel RW et al. Prospective randomized trial of polyglactin 910 mesh to prevent recurrence of cystoceles and rectoceles. American Journal of Obstetrics and Gynecology 2001; 184:1357–1362.

62. Young SB, Daman JJ, Bony LG. Vaginal paravaginal repair: one-year outcomes. American Journal of Obstetrics and Gynecology 2001; 185:1360–1366.

63. Shull BL, Benn SJ, Kuehl TJ. Surgical management of prolapse of the anterior vaginal segment: an analysis of support defects, operative morbidity, and anatomic outcome. American Journal of Obstetrics and Gynecology 1994; 171:1429–1436.

64. Haase P, Skibsted L. Influence of operations for stress incontinence and/or genital descensus on sexual life. Acta Obstetricia et Gynecologica Scandinavia 1988; 67:659–661.

65. Kahn MA, Stanton SL. Posterior colporrhaphy: its effects on bowel and sexual function. BJOG 1997; 104:82–86.

66. Kahn MA, Stanton SL. Techniques of rectocele repair and their effects on bowel function. International Urogynecology Journal 1998; 9:37–47.

67. Julian TM. The efficacy of Marlex mesh in the repair of severe, recurrent vaginal prolapse of the anterior midvaginal wall. American Journal of Obstetrics and Gynecology 1996; 175:1472–1475.

68. Milani R, Salvatore S, Soligo M et al. Functional and anatomical outcome of anterior and posterior vaginal prolapse repair with prolene mesh. BJOG 2005; 112:107–111.

69. Dwyer PL, O'Reilly BA. Transvaginal repair of anterior and posterior compartment prolapse with Atrium polypropylene mesh. BJOG 2004; 111:831–836.

70. Baessler K, Hewson AD, Tunn R et al. Severe mesh complications following intravaginal slingplasty. Obstetrics and Gynecology 2005; 106:713–716.

71. Bafghi A, Benizri EI, Trastour C et al. Multifilament polypropylene mesh for urinary incontinence: 10 cases of infections requiring removal of the sling. BJOG 2005; 112:376–378.

72. Chaliha C, Khalid U, Campagna L et al. SIS graft for anterior vaginal wall prolapse repair—a case-controlled study. International Urogynecology Journal 2006; 17:492–497.

73. Gandhi S, Goldberg RP, Kwon C et al. A prospective randomized trial using solvent dehydrated fascia lata for the prevention of recurrent anterior vaginal wall prolapse. American Journal of Obstetrics and Gynecology 2005; 192:1649–1654.

74. Denehy TR, Choe JY, Gregori CA et al. Modified Le Fort partial colpocleisis with Kelly urethral plication and posterior colpoperineoplasty in the medically compromised elderly: a comparison with vaginal hysterectomy, anterior colporrhaphy, and posterior colpoperineoplasty. American Journal of Obstetrics and Gynecology 1995; 173:1697–1702.

75. FitzGerald MP, Richter HE, Siddique S et al. Colpocleisis: a review. International Urogynecology Journal 2006; 17:261–271.

76. Barber MD, Amundsen CL, Paraiso MF et al. Quality of life after surgery for genital prolapse in elderly women: obliterative and reconstructive surgery. International Urogynecology Journal 2007; 18:799–806.

77. O'Boyle AL, Woodman PJ, O'Boyle JD et al. Pelvic organ support in nulliparous pregnant and nonpregnant women: a case control study. American Journal of Obstetrics and Gynecology 2002; 187:99–102.

78. O'Boyle AL, O'Boyle JD, Ricks RE et al. The natural history of pelvic organ support in pregnancy. International Urogynecology Journal 2003; 14:46–49.

10
Fecal Incontinence in Women

Joseph M. Novi
Department of Urogynecology and Reconstructive Pelvic Surgery,
Riverside Methodist Hospital, Columbus, Ohio, U.S.A.

I. INTRODUCTION

Fecal incontinence is a socially and psychologically distressing condition affecting a substantial number of women worldwide. The problem remains underreported and under treated. This is due, in part, to patients' and healthcare providers' reluctance to discuss the subject and lack of understanding of the pathophysiology and treatment options available. Paramount in the assessment of such patients is the history taking. It is incumbent upon the healthcare provider to actively question patients, since most patients with this problem will not offer the complaint of fecal incontinence.

II. DEFINITION

Fecal incontinence is defined as the involuntary passage of fecal material through the anal canal at any time after completion of toilet training. There are two subsets of fecal incontinence: complete and partial. Complete incontinence involves the loss of control of both liquid and solid feces and implies a more severe abnormality, while partial incontinence involves the loss of control of liquid stool or flatus.

III. PREVALENCE

The true prevalence of fecal incontinence is difficult to determine. The problem is socially and psychologically embarrassing and is therefore underreported. Johanson et al. found that only one-third of patients with fecal incontinence had ever discussed the problem with a physician (1). In a large mail survey of American households, 7.1% of the general population reported some degree of fecal incontinence (2). Among patients with urinary incontinence and pelvic organ prolapse, the prevalence of fecal incontinence is as high as 30% (3). An estimated 13% to 47% of hospitalized elderly patients and nursing home residents are affected (4,5). The female to male ratio is estimated to be 1.5:1 (6). Fecal incontinence is the second most common reason for institutionalization of the elderly and helps account for the greater than $400,000,000 per year spent on adult diapers in the United States (7).

IV. FECAL CONTINENCE MECHANISM

Anal continence is dependent upon the complex coordination of several muscles, intact neural pathways and cognition, distensibility of the rectum, and stool volume and consistency. The puborectalis portion of the levator ani musculature forms a sling-like band which originates on the pubic bone, passes alongside the vagina and fuses posterior to the rectum. It maintains a constant muscular tone, is responsible for the acute angulation of the anorectal junction, and helps maintain solid stool above the anal canal. At rest, the anorectal angle is approximately 90°, though with voluntary contraction of this muscle the angle may approach 70° (8). At the time of defecation, the puborectalis relaxes and the anorectal angle becomes more obtuse (110–130°), allowing stool to move into the anal canal.

The anal canal is normally closed at rest due to the constant tone of the internal anal sphincter (IAS) and external anal sphincter (EAS). The IAS is responsible for about 80% of the resting tone. Both the IAS and the EAS are involved in maintaining continence of liquid stool, with the EAS being the most important component.

Since the PR and IAS maintain constant tone, stool is normally stored above the anal canal. In response to distention of the rectum, the PR relaxes and allows some of the contents into the upper anal canal. As colonic contents enter the anal canal, the IAS relaxes and closure of the anus is largely due to EAS contraction. The sampling reflex occurs, allowing discrimination between solid or liquid stool and gas. If the external environment is not appropriate for defecation or the release of flatus, further contraction of the EAS and PR allows the IAS to regain tone, propelling the anal contents back into the rectum.

V. ETIOLOGY OF FECAL INCONTINENCE

Vaginal childbirth has long been recognized as a major contributor to the development of fecal incontinence (9). Injury to the internal and external anal sphincters sustained at the time of childbirth is the most frequent cause of incontinence (10). However, stretch and compression of the pudendal nerve, and damage of the levator ani musculature also play an important role. The uses of obstetric forceps and midline episiotomy have both been significantly associated with the development fecal incontinence (11–15). There have been mixed reports regarding fetal size greater than 4000 g, prolonged second stage of labor, and multiparity as etiologic factors for fecal incontinence, with some reports showing a significant association while others have not (16,17). Subsequent vaginal delivery in a woman with a previous anal sphincter injury has been associated with an increased risk of development of fecal incontinence (18,19). If a pregnant woman has a history of an anal sphincter injury in a previous pregnancy, some authors recommend the consideration of cesarean delivery, especially if the woman is currently continent (20,21).

Other iatrogenic causes of anal sphincter injury include anorectal surgeries such as fistulectomy/fistulotomy, hemorrhoidectomy, and, less commonly, lateral internal anal sphincterotomy for the treatment of chronic anal fissures (22). Appropriate care must be taken when performing fistula repairs, particularly those utilizing an anterior approach, to minimize injury to the anal sphincter complex.

The anal continence mechanism relies upon many factors working together to maintain proper function. The mucosa of the anus normally forms a hermetic seal, preventing the seepage of discharge. Circumstances that may impair the coaptation of the anal mucosa include full thickness rectal prolapse and protrusion of internal hemorrhoids. These conditions may allow the egress of mucus or liquid stool.

Neurologic factors play an important role in the continence mechanism. Motor and sensory function must be intact to maintain continence. Patients should be able to distinguish between gas, liquid, and solid stool (known as the sampling reflex) and be able to control anal sphincter musculature. Demyelinating diseases (e.g., multiple sclerosis), meningomyelocele, cauda equina syndrome, stroke, and spinal cord trauma are all associated with impairment of the anal sphincters. Patients with dementia, psychiatric conditions, or altered mentation may lack the awareness or motivation necessary to maintain continence.

Excessive amounts of stool may overwhelm even a normally functioning continence mechanism (23). Viral gastroenteritis, infectious colitis, chronic diarrheal states such as inflammatory bowel disease, irritable bowel syndrome, malabsorption, and laxative abuse may present abnormal volumes of solid and liquid stool to the anal canal. Since liquid stool in particular is more difficult to maintain than solid stool, overflow incontinence may occur. Alternatively, chronic constipation with straining can cause stretch injury and neuropathy of the pudendal nerve. If fecal impaction is present, prolonged reflex relaxation of the internal anal sphincter occurs, allowing liquid stool to bypass the impaction, leading to fecal soiling (24).

It is estimated that approximately 20% of diabetics experience some fecal incontinence (25,26). Most of these patients will have low-volume diarrhea and peripheral neuropathies. The causes of diarrhea in diabetics include autonomic dysfunction, pancreatic insufficiency, and bacterial overgrowth. However, since diarrhea in diabetics is low-volume, the presence of peripheral neuropathy has been postulated as the primary cause of incontinence in these patients (25,26). As opposed to fecal incontinence from other causes, fecal incontinence in diabetics is more prevalent in men than women (9).

Inflammation of the rectal mucosa due to radiation-induced proctitis, Crohn's colitis, and ulcerative colitis leads to extreme fecal urgency (27). Incontinence may occur if the patient cannot find a toilet soon after feeling the defecatory urge. Fecal incontinence associated with these syndromes is related to urgency, and is not a consequence of an anatomic sphincter abnormality. Since incontinence may be a presenting symptom of underlying gastrointestinal disease, it is important to uncover changes in bowel habits and institute an appropriate workup or referral.

Other causes of fecal incontinence include neoplasms, scleroderma, sexual abuse, and anal intercourse (9). Neoplasms may cause a functional obstruction and lead to fecal soiling similar to that seen with fecal impaction. Scleroderma affects smooth muscle more than striated muscle. Internal anal sphincter pressures are lower in these patients, while external anal sphincter pressures may be normal (28). Although these are difficult subjects to discuss with patients, all patients should be screened for sexual abuse as part of the routine history taking, and the sexual history should include questions related to anal intercourse.

VI. EVALUATION

The evaluation starts with taking a thorough history. Questions should focus on elucidating the duration of the problem, the frequency of incontinence, the use of protective pads/diapers, frequency of bowel movements, constipation, diarrhea, rectal bleeding/discharge (possibly indicative of neoplasm or inflammatory bowel conditions), and laxative abuse. The quality of stool lost (solid or liquid) as well as the ability to control flatus should be ascertained to help judge the severity of the problem (flatus is more difficult to control than liquid stool; solid stool is easiest to control). Attempts should be made to distinguish fecal urgency from incontinence, as urgency may reflect an inability of the rectum to store stool rather than a defect in the sphincter complex. A complaint of fecal urgency should prompt a mucosal evaluation to rule out neoplasms and inflammatory bowel disease (see below). The patient should also be questioned regarding the effects of incontinence on their daily life, and any changes they have made to accommodate the incontinence.

The medical/surgical history should include questions about previous back injuries/surgeries, cancers, irradiation, diabetes, multiple sclerosis, scleroderma, psychiatric problems, bowel diseases, neurologic diseases, and anorectal and abdominal surgeries.

The ob/gyn history focuses on the number and type of deliveries (cesarean birth vs. spontaneous vaginal delivery vs. operative vaginal delivery), episiotomy, perineal lacerations and/or infections, and birth weights. A complete sexual history, including abuse and anal intercourse, should be determined.

VII. PHYSICAL EXAMINATION

The physical exam of a patient complaining of fecal incontinence should include all of the following parameters:

-   Pelvic exam with evaluation of pelvic organ prolapse (done in the supine and standing positions), assessment for masses, and pelvic floor muscle strength
-   Neurologic exam including gait, anocutaneous reflex (sacral reflex arc), and lower extremity sensory and motor function
-   Inspection of perianal area for scars, fissures, hemorrhoids, skin irritation, mucosal prolapse, gaping anus, and perianal creases
-   Digital rectal exam to assess resting tone, masses, fecal impaction, occult blood
-   Inspection of undergarments for soiling
-   Upright exam—straining on commode to demonstrate rectal prolapse (if indicated)

VIII. DIAGNOSTIC TESTING

The diagnostic work-up of a patient with fecal incontinence should be tailored to the individual patient. Every patient will not need each of the tests described.

A. Mucosal Evaluation

The patient with fecal urgency, rectal bleeding, stool positive for occult blood, and/or a change in bowel habits should undergo proctosigmoidoscopy to evaluate for inflammatory conditions and tumors (10). Referral to a gastroenterologist or colorectal surgeon should be considered.

B. Enema

If the history and physical exam remain ambiguous, an enema may help determine whether or not a patient is truly having incontinence. One hundred milliliters of tap water is instilled into rectum and the patient is asked to hold this for a few minutes. If the patient can maintain water in the rectum, she probably does not have significant incontinence since liquid is more difficult to control than stool (29).

A variation of the enema test is the saline infusion test. It has been suggested as both an evaluation tool and an objective method of assessing clinical improvement after therapy (30). With the patient in the supine position, a 2-mm tube is placed into the rectum a distance of 10 cm and then secured with tape. The patient is then transferred to a commode. The tube is attached to an infusion pump that delivers warm (body temperature) saline at a rate of 60 ml/min up to a total of 1500 ml. The patient is asked to hold the liquid in the rectum for as long as possible. During filling, the volume at first onset of leakage (defined as at least 25 ml) and the total volume remaining in the rectum at the end of the test are recorded. Patients with a normally functioning continence mechanism should be able to retain most of the liquid in the rectum, while women with fecal incontinence will leak at much lower volumes (31,32).

C. Stool Culture

Particularly for patients with diarrhea, or who have taken antibiotics within the past six months, a stool culture may be warranted to rule out an infectious etiology (33).

D. Anorectal Manometry

Anorectal manometry measures both resting tone (internal anal sphincter) and squeeze pressure (external anal sphincter). The functional length of the anal canal can be determined by the measured distance of these pressures. This test is particularly useful in evaluating sphincter trauma, such as anterior injury due to obstetric trauma. Also, it can provide an assessment of rectal sensation and compliance which may aid in predicting surgical outcomes (34).

E. Defecography

Dynamic radiologic evaluation of the rectum (defecography) has a very limited role in the investigation of fecal incontinence. It may be helpful if pelvic organ prolapse and/or rectal prolapse is suspected but cannot be demonstrated on physical exam (29). It is particularly useful in detecting an enterocele.

F. Endoanal Ultrasound

A specialized ultrasound probe, capable of acquiring images in a 360° view, is inserted into the rectum and images are obtained upon withdrawal. The internal anal sphincter appears as an innermost hypoechoic area and the external anal sphincter is hyperechoic (Fig. 1). Currently, it is the test of choice for defining the anatomy of the anal sphincters and should be performed only if surgical repair is contemplated. The information obtained from these images will assist in preoperative surgical planning (29).

G. Magnetic Resonance Imaging (MRI)

MRI is currently being investigated as a diagnostic tool for fecal incontinence. It is the only imaging method that can visualize the anal sphincters and movement of the pelvic floor musculature without radiation exposure. Though MRI has been shown to be more accurate at identifying external anal sphincter abnormalities than ultrasound, its use is limited by availability, cost, and lack of normative data in asymptomatic patients (35).

H. Nerve Conduction Studies

Pudendal nerve terminal motor latency (PNTML) is a measure of the conduction velocity across the distal part of the nerve. A gloved finger with an electrode attached to the tip of the glove is inserted into the anal canal and used to stimulate the pudendal nerve. The impulse is detected and the latency period measured using surface electrodes on the perineum. If prolonged conduction times are noted, this may be evidence of impaired nerve input to the anal sphincters and puborectalis muscle. This test is mainly used in the preoperative assessment of patients considering sphincter repair, as the results may be helpful in predicting the success of the repair. However, some studies have failed to show that nerve prolongation negatively affects surgical results, (36) while others show normal conduction to be a predictor of favorable outcomes (37). Additionally, in patients with idiopathic fecal incontinence, normal PNTML does not exclude weakness of the pelvic floor (37).

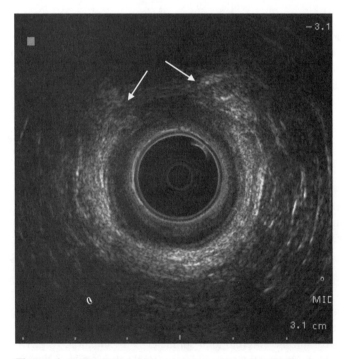

Figure 1 External anal sphincter appears hyperechoic. The arrows are pointing to the ends of the disrupted external anal sphincter. The internal anal sphincter is the hypoechoic structure medial to the external anal sphincter.

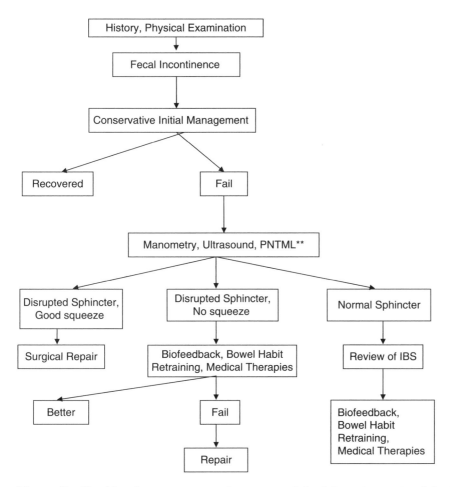

Figure 2 Algorithm for assessment and treatment of fecal incontinence in adults. Pudendal nerve terminal motor latency testing. *Source:* Adapted from the International Continence Society Recommendations (61).

IX. TREATMENT

Treatment should be directed to the underlying cause. Preliminary surgical treatments may include cancer resection, repair of rectal prolapse, treatment of inflammatory bowel disease, and removal of impactions.

X. NONSURGICAL THERAPIES

A. Scheduled Toileting

Ritualizing bowel habits may prove of significant value, especially in the institutionalized patient. Scheduled toileting allows the patient to evacuate the lower bowel, possibly reducing episodes of incontinence due to the inability of staff and/or the patient to quickly respond to fecal urgency. Additionally, a scheduled morning enema may also reduce the likelihood of incontinence episodes by reducing the amount of stool in the lower bowel.

B. Dietary Modifications

Caffeine has been shown to increase colonic motility and augment fluid secretion in the small intestine. Reduction of caffeine may reduce fecal urgency and result in firmer stools. A food and symptom diary may reveal lactose and/or fructose intolerance. Avoidance of these dietary substances in patients demonstrating intolerance should improve fecal incontinence symptoms (38).

C. Medical Therapies

Bulking agents, such as Metamucil, Citracel, or Konsyl, can change the consistency of the stool, making it firmer and more easily controlled. Daily enemas help to keep the rectum free of stool. With the addition of bulking agents to the enema regimen, it may reduce the incidence of stooling in between desired defecation.

Agents to slow motility of the intestinal tract can help by slightly constipating patients, allowing them to better control their stool. Loperamide hydrochloride prolongs intestinal transit time, allowing fecal volume to be reduced. The increased transit time allows for additional removal of fluid from the stool, and the bulk density to increase. Loperamide also increases rectal compliance, which decreases urgency. In several clinical trials, loperamide was shown to significantly reduce stool frequency and urgency, increase colonic transit time, reduce stool weight, and increase resting anal sphincter tone compared to placebo (39–41).

Diphenoxylate hydrochloride is another agent used to increase intestinal transit time, especially if diarrhea is the major reason for the incontinence. It is less expensive than loperamide, but is a Schedule V drug and has a minimal potential for physical dependence.

D. Pelvic Floor Exercises

There are no studies that show a definite improvement in fecal incontinence with a regimen of pelvic floor muscle-strengthening exercises. Since they are safe and without cost, they should be discussed with patients affected with fecal incontinence. A trained physical therapist may help to optimize results.

E. Biofeedback

Several studies have demonstrated a significant improvement in fecal incontinence with biofeedback (42,43). Improvement rates of 63% to 90% have been reported (43). Additionally, Jensen and Lowry showed that biofeedback improved outcomes after sphincteroplasty (44). Unfortunately, it is labor-intensive and requires a dedicated therapist. Biofeedback involves placing a balloon in the rectum to simulate stool. Anal sphincter contraction is measured with a second balloon or perineal surface electrodes. Visual feedback provides direct encouragement when proper sphincter response is made. Gradually, the volume is decreased and patients learn to sense smaller volumes in the rectum while increasing control of the anal sphincter. In 2004, Palsson et al. performed a review of the literature on the efficacy of biofeedback for functional anorectal disorders (45). They concluded that "biofeedback treatment may therefore be viewed as a valuable adjunct to medical management of incontinence."

F. Clitoral Stimulation

Stimulation of sensory nerve endings has been shown to improve motor function of the same nerve, and serves as the basis for clitoral stimulation and its effect on pudendal nerve function (46). One small trial (39 women) reported a significant decrease in incontinence symptom scores and improvement in anal sphincter tone after eight weeks of therapy (47). Larger studies with longer-term follow-up are necessary to better evaluate this treatment modality.

XI. SURGICAL THERAPIES

A. Anal Sphincteroplasty

When an anatomic defect in the anal sphincter complex is identified, surgical correction is a viable option. Ideally, at least three to six months should elapse after the injury to allow inflammation to subside prior to attempting surgical repair. Sphincteroplasty is the mainstay of operative repair. The internal sphincter should be identified and repaired along its entire length, which is approximately 3 cm to 4 cm. The external sphincter is then identified and reapproximated. There have been conflicting reports of outcomes comparing end-to-end repair versus overlapping repair of the external anal sphincter (34,49). The important concepts are to mobilize a sufficient length of muscle to affect a tension-free repair, and to use long-acting absorbable suture, such as polydiaxanone (PDS, Ethicon, Somerville, N.J.) or polyglyconate (Maxon, U.S. Surgical, Norwalk, C.T.). Unfortunately, though short-term results are good, long-term studies of patients after spincteroplasty have been disappointing, with 5- and 10-year success rates less than 40% (49,50).

B. Dynamic Graciloplasty

Dynamic graciloplasty involves transposing the gracilis muscle from the inner thigh to wrap around the anal canal, attaching the tendon to the contralateral ischial tuberosity, and then stimulating the muscle to maintain constant tone. The stimulator is placed subcutaneously in the abdominal wall. Leads are then threaded subcutaneously and attached to stimulating electrodes placed in the muscle close to the nerve supply. Success rates have been reported in the 70% to 82% range (48). However, in a recent report of long-term follow-up (five years), only 16% of patients with a functioning dynamic graciloplasty had normal fecal continence (51). In this same study, 72% of patients had pain, swelling, or paresthesia of the donor leg, 27% had sexual dysfunction, and 16% had been converted to an end-colostomy for persistent incontinence.

C. Artificial Bowel Sphincter

The artificial bowel sphincter is designed to replace the anal sphincter for the treatment of severe refractory fecal incontinence. The artificial bowel sphincter has been adapted from the artificial urinary sphincter and involves the placement of an inflatable cuff around the anal canal. A pump that inflates and deflates the artificial bowel sphincter is placed in the labium majus. A balloon reservoir is placed in the retroperitoneal space superior to the bladder. The pump is activated, inflating the cuff and closing the anal canal. When the patient desires to defecate, the pump deflates the cuff by transferring the fluid to the balloon reservoir. Success rates are reported in the 49% to 60% range, with infection rates of 19% to 34%. Incontinence severity scores were significantly improved in those patients who had successful artificial bowel sphincter placement, and the function appears to remain stable more than two years after surgery (52).

D. Sacral Nerve Stimulation

Sacral nerve stimulation involves the placement of electrodes through the S2, S3, or S4 sacral foramen to provide stimulation of the pelvic floor muscles. This technique is reserved for patients who have intact sphincters that are functionally deficient. A test stimulator may be used to determine which patients are the best candidates for a permanent implant. The permanent stimulator is placed subcutaneously in the abdominal wall and connected to the electrodes via subcutaneously threaded leads. Several studies have shown improved resting and squeeze anal sphincter pressures, and improved rectal sensation (53–55). However, the mechanism of action remains uncertain. Possible theories include stimulation of sensory afferents, stimulation of motor afferents, and modulation of neural reflexes (56). Though published series have reported on a small number of patients, the significant improvement in incontinence episodes has been demonstrated in 70% to 80% of patients with minimal morbidity (57,58).

E. Colostomy/Ileostomy

Fecal diversion, with colostomy or ileostomy, may provide significant relief in patients who have failed other invasive therapies or are not candidates for anal sphincter replacement. This option may allow patients trapped at home by fear of embarrassment to lead a more normal social life.

F. Radiofrequency Ablation

One of the promising new treatments for fecal incontinence is radio frequency ablation. Using conscious sedation and local anesthesia, temperature-controlled radio frequency energy is delivered via an anoscopic device with multiple needle electrodes to create thermal lesions deep to the mucosa of the anal canal, (59) creating scarring and narrowing of the anal canal and retraction of the anal sphincter complex. This modality has been used in a small number of patients but has been shown to significantly reduce symptoms and improve quality of life scores (60). Further studies are needed to validate the long-term success of this procedure.

XII. CONCLUSION

Fecal incontinence is a devastating condition for both patients and their care-givers. It can have a major impact on the quality of life of those patients who are afflicted. Many therapeutic options exist for the treatment of fecal incontinence, but identifying affected patients remains an elusive and important first-step in the evaluation process.

REFERENCES

1. Johanson JF, Lafferty J. Epidemiology of fecal incontinence: the silent affliction. Am J Gastroenterol 1996; 91(1):33–36.
2. Drossman DA, Li Z, Andruzzi E et al. U.S. householder survey of functional gastroeneterologic disorders. Dig Dis Sci 1993; 38:1569–1580.

3. Eva UF, Gun W, Preben K. Prevalence of urinary and fecal incontinence and symptoms of genital prolapse in women. Acta Obstet Gynecol Scand 2003; 82:280–286.

4. Tobin GW, Brocklehurst JC. Faecal incontinence in residential homes for the elderly: Prevalence, aetiology and management. Age Ageing 1986; 15(1):41–46.

5. Clarke M. Hughes AO, Dodd KJ et al. The elderly in residential care: Patterns of disability. Health Trends 1979; 11:17–20.

6. Nelson R, Norton N, Cautley E et al. Community-based prevalence of anal incontinence. JAMA 1995; 274:559–561.

7. Jorge JM, Wexner SD. Etiology and management of fecal incontinence. Dis Colon Rectum 1993; 36:77–97.

8. Rao SSC. Diagnosis and management of fecal incontinence. Am J Gastroenterol 2004; 99(8):1585–1604.

9. Cooper ZR, Rose S. Fecal incontinence: A clinical approach. Mt Sinai J Med 2000; 67(2): 96–105.

10. Rudolph W, Galandiuk S. A Practical guide to the diagnosis and management of fecal incontinence. Mayo Clin Proc 2002; 77(3):271–275.

11. MacArthur C, Glazener CM, Wilson PD et al. Obstetric practice and faecal incontinence three months after delivery. BJOG 2001; 108(7):678–683.

12. Signorello LB, Harlow BL, Chekos AK et al. Midline episiotomy and anal incontinence: retrospective cohort study. BMJ 200; 320:86–90.

13. DeLeeuw JW, Vierhout ME, Struijk PC et al. Anal sphincter damage after vaginal delivery: functional outcome and risk factors for fecal incontinence. Acta Obstet Gynecol Scand 2001; 80:830–834.

14. Meyer S, Hohlfeld P, Achtari C et al. Birth trauma: short- and long-term effects of forceps delivery compared with spontaneous delivery on various pelvic floor parameters. BJOG 2000; 107(11):1360–1365.

15. Toglia MR, DeLancey JOL. Anal incontinence and the obstetrician-gynecologist. Obstet Gynecol 1994; 84(4):731–740.

16. Abramowitz L, Sobhani I, Ganansia R et al. Are sphincter defects the cause of anal incontinence after vaginal delivery? Results of a prospective study. Dis Colon Rectum 2000; 43(5):590–596.

17. Eason E, Labrecque M, Marcoux S et al. Anal incontinence after childbirth. CMAJ 2002; 166(3):326–336.

18. Sangalli MR, Floris L, Faltin D et al. Anal incontinence in women with third or fourth degree perineal tears and subsequent vaginal deliveries. Aust N Z J Obstet Gynaecol 2000; 40(3):244–248.

19. Faltin DL, Sangalli MR, Roche B et al. Does a second delivery increase the risk of anal incontinence? BJOG 2001 108(7):684–688.

20. Faridi A, Willis S, Schelzig P et al. Anal sphincter injury during vaginal delivery—an argument for cesarean on request? J Perinat Med 2002; 30(5):379–387.

21. McKenna DS, Ester JB, Fischer JR. Elective cesarean delivery for women with a previous anal sphincter rupture. Am J Obstet Gynecol 2003; 189:1251–1256.

22. Zbar AP, Beer-Gabel M, Chiappa AC et al. Fecal incontinence after minor anorectal surgery. Dis Colon Rectum 2001; 44(11):1610–1619.

23. Herbst F, Kamm MA, Morris GP et al. Gastrointestinal transit and prolonged ambulatory colonic motility in health and faecal incontinence. Gut 1997; 41:381–389.

24. Read NW, Abouzekry L, Read MG et al. Anorectal function in elderly patients with fecal impaction. Gastroenterology 1985; 89:959–966.

25. Schiller LR, Santa Ana CA, Schulmen AC et al. Pathogenesis of fecal incontinence in diabetes mellitus: Evidence for internal-anal-sphincter dysfunction. N Engl J Med 1982; 307: 1666–1671.

26. Caruana BJ, Wald A. Hinds JP et al. Anorectal sensory and motor function in neurogenic fecal incontinence. Gastroenterology 1991; 100:465–470.

27. Rao SSC, Read NW, Davison P et al. Anorectal sensitivity and responses to rectal distention in patients with ulcerative colitis. Gastroenterology 1987; 93:1020–1026.

28. Jaffin BW, Chang P, Spiera H. Fecal incontinence in scleroderma. Clinical features, anorectal manometric findings and their therapeutic implications. J Clin Gastroenterol 1997; 25(3):513–517.

29. Hull TL. Fecal Incontinence. In Urogynecology and Reconstructive Pelvic Surgery, Second Edition. Karram M, Walters MD, eds. Mosby, Philadelphia; 1999:259–268.

30. Rao SSC, Happel J, Welcher K. Can biofeedback therapy improve anorectal function in fecal incontinence? Am J Gastroenterol 1996; 91:2360–2366.

31. Rao SSC. Manometric evaluation of defecation disorders, Part II: Fecal incontinence. The Gastroenterologist 1997; 5(2):99–111.

32. Rao SSC, Hatfield R, Leistikow J et al. Manometric tests of anorectal function in healthy humans. Am J Gastroenterol 1999; 94:773–783.

33. Soffer EE, Hull T. Fecal incontinence: A practical approach to evaluation and treatment. AJG 2000; 95(8):1873–1880.

34. Young CJ, Mathur MN, Eyers AA et al. Successful overlapping anal sphincter repair: Relationship to patient age, neuropathy, and colostomy formation. Dis Colon Rectum 1998; 41:344–349.

35. Rociu E, Stoker J, Eijkemans MJ et al. Fecal incontinence: endoanal US versus endoanal MR imaging. Radiology 1999; 212:453–458.

36. Gilliland R, Altomare DF, Moreira H et al. Pudendal nerve neuropathy is predictive of failure following anterior sphincteroplasty. Dis Colon Rectum 1998; 41:1516–1522.

37. Suilleabhain CB, Horgan AF, McEnroe L. The relationship of pudendal nerve terminal motor latency to squeeze pressure in patients with idiopathic fecal incontinence. Dis Colon Rectum 2001; 44(5):666–671.

38. Choi YK, Johlin FC Jr, Summers RW et al. Fructose intolerance: an under-recognized problem. Am J Gastroenterol 2003; 98:1348–1353.

39. Sun WM, Read NW, Verlinden M. Effects of loperamide oxide on gastrointestinal transit time and anorectal function in patients with chronic diarrhea and faecal incontinence. Scand J Gastroenterol 1997; 32:34–38.

40. Hallgren T, Fasth S, Delbro DS et al. Loperamide improves anal sphincter function and continence after restorative protocolectomy. Dig Dis Sci 1994; 39:2612–2618.

41. Harford WV, Krejs GJ, Santa Ana CA et al. Acute effect of diphenoxylate with atropine (Lomotil) in patients with chronic diarrhea and fecal incontinence. Gastroenterology 1980; 78:440–443.

42. Jorge JM, Habr-Gama A, Wexner SD. Biofeedback therapy in the colon and rectal practice. Appl Psychophysiol Biofeedback 2003; 28(1):47–61.

43. Solomon MJ, Pager CK, Rex J et al. Randomized, controlled trial of biofeedback with anal manometry, transanal ultrasound, or pelvic floor retraining with digital guidance alone in the treatment of mild to moderate fecal incontinence. Dis Colon Rectum 2003; 46(6):703–710.

44. Arnaud A, Sarles JC, Sielezneff I et al. Sphincter repair without overlapping for fecal incontinence. Dis Colon Rectum 1996; 34:744–747.

45. Palsson OS, Heyman S, Whitehead WE. Biofeedback treatment for functional anorectal disorders: A comprehensive efficacy review. Appl Psychophysiol Biofeedback 2004; 29(3):153–174.

46. Brindley GS. Treatment of urinary and faecal incontinence by surgically implanted devices. Ciba Foundation Symp 1990; 151:267–274.

47. Frizelle FA, Gearry RB, Johnston M et al. Penile and clitoral stimulation for faecal incontinence: external application of a bipolar electrode for patients with faecal incontinence. Colorectal Dis 2004; 6(1):54–57.

48. Rongen MJ, Uludag O, El Naggar K et al. Long-term follow-up of dynamic graciloplasty for fecal incontinence. Dis Colon Rectum 2003; 46(6):716–721.

49. Gutierrez B, Madoff RD, Lowry AC et al. Long-term results of anterior sphincteroplasty. Dis Colon Rectum 2004; 47(5):727–731.

50. Halverson AL, Hull TL. Long-term outcome of overlapping anal sphincter repair. Dis Colon Rectum 2002; 45:345–348.

51. Thornton MJ, Kennedy ML, Lubowski DZ et al. Long-term follow-up of dynamic graciloplasty for faecal incontinence. Colorectal Dis 2004; 6:470–476.

52. Parker SC, Spencer MP, Madoff RD et al. Artificial bowel sphincter: long-term experience at a single institution. Dis Colon Rectum 2003; 46(6):722–729.

53. Kenefick NJ, Vaizey CJ, Cohen RC et al. Medium-term results of permanent sacral nerve stimulation for faecal incontinence. Br J Surg 2002; 89(7):896–901.

54. Matzel KE, Stadelmaier U, Hohenfellner M et al. Chronic sacral spinal nerve stimulation for fecal incontinence: long-term results with foramen and cuff electrodes. Dis Colon Rectum 2001; 44:59–66.

55. Leroi AM, Michot F, Grise P et al. Effect of sacral nerve stimulation in patients with faecal and urinary incontinence. Dis Colon Rectum 2001; 44:779–789.

56. Madoff RD. Surgical treatment options for fecal incontinence. Gastroenterology 2004; 126(1):S48–S54.

57. Uludag O, Koch SM, van Gemert WG et al. Sacral neuromodulation in patients with fecal incontinence: a single-center study. Dis Colon Rectum 2004; 47(8):1350–1357.

58. Rosen HR, Urbarz C, Holzer B et al. Sacral nerve stimulation as a treatment for fecal incontinence. Gastroenterology 2001; 121:536–541.

59. Takahashi T, Garcia-Osogobio S, Valdovinos MA et al. Radio-frequency energy delivery to the anal canal for the treatment of fecal incontinence. Dis Colon Rectum 2002; 45(7):915–922.

60. Takahashi T, Garcia-Osogobio S, Valdovinos MA et al. Extended two-year results of radio-frequency energy delivery for the treatment of fecal incontinence (the Secca procedure). Dis Colon Rectum 2003; 46(6):711–715.

61. Norton C, Christiansen J, Butler U et al. International Continence Society Committee on Anal Incontinence Recommendations, 2001.

Index

Page references followed by f indicate an illustrative figure; t indicate a table